Magpie

A Novella

by

Mark W. Lyon

Dedication

With faith and humor

John Goldenberg showed me the path.

Dr. Stephen Weil encouraged me to walk.

Contents

Prologue

This driver is going to kill us.

Reynaud sweat in the passenger seat, his body twisting with fear. *We will crash. I will die in the desert.*

For three hours, he'd been trapped in a race to hell. His eyes ached from tension as he stared out the windshield, watching the SUV swallow white lines on the asphalt and teeter on the edge of destruction around every curve of the highway from Jedda.

Now long past sundown, the day's stifling heat lingered in the interior like an ill-mannered guest. In spite of this, Reynaud sat rigid in a suit and tie. He closed his eyes, but that only heightened his other discomforts: tires roared in his ears, perspiration itched down his body into his crotch, a barnyard smell emanated from the sheep herder slouched in the back seat.

He opened his eyes and stared again through the grimy windshield at a spot on the horizon where the two rows of mercury vapor lamps above the four-lane highway converged, at the evil waiting there.

He flicked his eyes left and stole a look at the driver, calm in his crisp desert camo, rushing them to the grave. One wrist draped over the steering wheel. The crystal on his huge watch flashed with every streetlight that whizzed overhead.

Reynaud glanced at his own sweaty hands, white knuckles clutching the stained leather briefcase on his lap as if gripping his terror-stricken heart.

He felt sudden movement near his left shoulder and a flush of barnyard reek in his nose. From the rear seat, the swarthy farmer, Nazih, leaned forward and thrust one hand across the driver's face toward the left side of the highway.

"Here. The turn is here," Nazih shouted.

The driver glared at Nazih, a hostile rebuke to let him know the instruction was late. Then he stomped the brakes.

The SUV skidded, stopped. Renaud slid into the footwell. The driver slammed into reverse. The transmission whined and they veered backward to the turnoff.

Then, with no hint of irritation, he shifted gently into first and fishtailed onto the rough dirt track. Reynaud struggled to regain his seat and again stared out the windshield, eyes wide, clutching his case.

"Sheep herder," snapped the driver. "How far?"

"A short walk," Nazih's only frame of reference. "Soon."

~

In the desert of Al Akhal, Abbas Mohammed al Surryah sat cross-legged on the warm sand. He sucked the grease from the calloused fingers of his right hand. Tasted the last dregs of lamb scooped from the tin plate in his lap.

There was no wind this evening. The sheep herder watched his two young sons chase each other in the flickering light of the cook fire. His ears confirmed that the horses had established themselves behind the tent. The camels, settled on their knees beside an ancient Datsun pickup, would belch and chew through the night. He heard the sheep. *Why were they moving?*

"Jameel." The father's Arabic was quiet, but firm. "Take your brother. Go to the sheep. See what is the trouble." The boys halted their game and raced into the twilight, their obedience a source of wonder and joy to the young father.

Abbas stood and carried his plate toward the tent, but stopped when he heard the rumble of an approaching vehicle. The sound explained the restless sheep. In the distance, he saw a glow of headlights bounce over the road. Watched them speed toward him.

Soon, a loam-streaked SUV plowed to a stop beside the Datsun and sent the livestock lumbering from the commotion and swirling dust. Abbas was relieved when his cousin Nazih leapt from the vehicle.

"Abbas. The doctor is here."

Finally, thought the sheep herder and he started for the SUV. He froze when he heard his wife wail from the tent.

"Nashwa, Nashwa," she cried. "Abbas, help!"

He ran for the tent, still clutching the tin plate.

Abbas halted inside the tent's main room and saw Farah in the lantern's soft light. She was hunched over, wringing her hands, looking down at Nashwa, their seven-year-old daughter, who lay on a tattered rug, wrapped in a woolen blanket.

They were not in the Muharram, the women's room, but that didn't surprise him. She expected the doctor.

Abbas ignored Farah and knelt beside the girl. He frowned when he saw her drawn face, black eyes, and the streaks of dried blood discharged from her nose and mouth.

"Abbas," sobbed Farah, "She is worse. I—I don't know what to do."

Angrily, Abbas flung the plate. She ducked and it sailed into a corner. Nazih cleared his throat in the doorway and Abbas nodded for him to enter. Nazih saw Farah and hesitated, looked again at Abbas, who motioned for his cousin to join him in the dim space.

Abbas didn't like the arrogant look of the driver who strutted behind Nazah. He saw the doctor holding a briefcase to his chest and sniffing the air like a frightened dog. The man wrinkled his nose and stepped awkwardly to the sheep herder's side. Abbas made room for the thin man and watched him kneel, place the briefcase precisely on the rug, and remove a small light from a pocket inside his suit coat.

He hadn't seen many doctors before. This one moved with

purpose: He barely touched his daughter. Rolled her gently, silently examined her eyes and ears. Pressed her belly through the wool blanket. He opened the briefcase and grabbed a notebook and pen. The doctor kept his head down, watched his hands write in the book. Finally, he spoke.

"From which animals does she drink milk?" he asked in French. The driver translated.

"Camels," Abbas responded in Arabic. "We have no goats." He watched the driver translate.

"I saw these symptoms some days ago in Jedda," Reynaud said without looking up. "A butcher. Sheep's blood got into cuts on his hand."

When the driver finished translating, Farah wailed.

Abbas kept his eyes on Reynaud, but commanded Farah to silence with a sharp chop of his hand.

"I have sheep, but she never touches blood," he told the driver, who translated.

"Good," said Reynaud. "The butcher died. Insha'Allah, your daughter will do better."

Indicium

Doctor Anders van der Veer, a fit twenty-eight year old, felt the Italian marble, cool on his feet, as he leaned over one of the bathroom sinks in his exclusive Pacific Heights home. The tall Dutchman was wrapped in a towel, shaving in his gold-framed mirror. Her mirror, an identical twin over the room's other sink, reflected no one.

The emptiness in the room bothered him less than the emptiness in his heart. She had left a year ago, but he still felt abandoned. His fault or not, it didn't matter. He was lonely. He fantasized that Pryia was there. In the mirror he saw her behind him. She leaned over his shoulder and scowled.

"You lied!" her accusation. He heard it.

Anders shut his eyes and clenched them tight for as long as he could, trying to obliterate the image, the guilt. When he finally peeked, she was gone. He exhaled, set the razor on the sink. Made himself take a dozen more deep breaths. When he felt his pulse slow, he picked up the razor and finished shaving. Pryia's sudden appearance in the mirror turned his thoughts to the woman who had darted in and out of his fantasies. Not his wife. The one he couldn't let go.

Twenty minutes later, Anders stood dressed for work at the granite counter in the kitchen. He'd just spilled a few drops of his

French-press Arabian dark roast coffee. When he reached for a dish cloth to wipe it up, he imagined the sound of clumsy footfalls and looked warily at the door to the garage.

Pryia, in her raincoat, wrestled an overstuffed suitcase out the door. She slammed it against the frame and down three steps onto the concrete. A hand reached back through the opening and pulled the door shut with a bang.

Anders dropped the dish cloth, put his palms on the granite, leaned into the counter, and bowed his head. He'd felt it before. Once the guilt started, he never knew when it would end.

Another ten minutes. His spirits had not improved. He carried his briefcase through the same door to the garage. He walked to the BMW loaner, opened the driver side door, and flung his briefcase across the interior onto the passenger seat. He ducked his head and dropped into the driver's seat, slammed the door and waited to catch his breath. Calm himself. Then he started the engine and pulled onto the street.

He'd gone as far as the traffic light on Van Ness and Broadway before he felt her next to him. He glanced right, straight into her blazing eyes.

"All those years and this is how you repay me."

He finally lost it.

"My God, Priya! Will you stop? I made a mistake. I apologized. I begged your forgiveness. I am in agony. What else can I do? You haunting me every waking moment does not help!"

That felt better. At least she had disappeared—for now.

~

When first-time patients step out of the elevator into the tiny reception of the San Francisco Fertility Clinic, they usually experience an overwhelming sensation of peace, an island of calm in a building that housed a busy hospital. The clinic was one of the first and was still one of the most highly regarded reproductive centers in the world. It was known to coax healthy babies from infertile couples where others had failed. A reputation based on the success of its founding partner, Doctor Anders van der Veer, in pioneering new methods to enhance fertility.

Seated at a small table, almost hidden among the lush plants and inviting chairs, a receptionist in her mid-twenties, Amy Jenkins, greeted all visitors with a heartfelt smile.

This morning, she noticed something different as Anders approached her station. His surgical cap, mask, and the gown embroidered with his name were his usual garb, but his body language was withdrawn. She knew he'd been unhappy for months but today it seemed more than normal.

"Amy, has the dealer delivered my car yet?"

"No Doctor. I will call them again."

He towered over her for a moment, tentative.

"What about my wife? Don't suppose—"

There it was. The ritual. She looked away from his listless eyes.

"No. I'm sorry."

Anders kept to his part of the tableau and walked away. His despondence had almost caused her to fumble her mental calendar, but she recovered and called after him.

"Oh, uh, Doctor. Rudy wants to see you right away in the lab."

She watched him walk away and nod to indicate he had understood and then his shoulders bunched up beneath his lab coat.

Anders took the stairs two at a time to the floor above, hurried to the Analysis Lab, and opened the door. His assistant, Rudy, was in a world of his own, facing away from the door at a lab table cluttered with oscilloscopes, meters, and glass tubes. He bounced back and forth on his feet and Anders thought he might sprint to the nearest urinal at any second. The twenty-five-year-old had a speed habit that didn't hinder his brilliant work. Anders tolerated it. He stepped close behind his pet bundle of nerves and stopped, peered down over his shoulder.

"Rudy, whatcha got?"

Whenever Rudy tried to suppress his agitation, he overcompensated. He turned suddenly and threw up his hands, startling Anders.

"At last! You're here!" He pointed at several prints lying on the lab bench. "Look. See this?"

Rudy's hands skittered over the table and positioned two of the pages side-by-side. Three graphs were printed, one above the other, across the width of each page. In each panel a series of nine sharp peaks rose at varied intervals like a line of jagged mountains.

Rudy snatched a pen from his lab coat pocket and jabbed back and forth between the two pages at the spikes in each panel to show Anders where they were different.

"Rudy, slow down."

"Okay. From the gene markers here and here." He pointed to the graphs and eyed Anders with a triumphant look. "Davidson children? Not from their parents."

Anders straightened. "Cannot be," he stammered. "I did their procedures myself." His pitch rose. "Julia took blood from the entire family while they were in my office."

"The Davidson's original home kit tested only the father. I tested the Y-Chromosome DNA from the father and also the mitochondrial DNA from the mother. Of the fifteen markers, we had twelve exclusions from the father and eleven from the mother. With only three exclusions we would report that parent and child are not related."

"I still don't buy it."

"Wait." Rudy shoved the printouts aside and slid three similar ones to the center of the table.

"Now, look." His pen indicated the identical positions of spikes in all of the pages. "Here, here, and here." He grew even more animated and stabbed the printouts repeatedly to emphasize his words.

"These are the Davidson twins. This is the Menendez kid. We got better than a 99.9 percent probability that they are siblings."

Anders glanced around as if he'd lost something. "No way, unless they're from the same mother."

"Yeah. And I tested the Philips kid from Chicago. He's a match, too."

"That's a lot of mother."

"Somebody screw up in the lab?"

"Rudy, please."

"What about when Theresa dropped a petri dish with the embryos—"

Anders felt a sharp ping in his right temple. He shook his head.

"Yeah, but the odds against something like this?" Rudy insisted.

"Astronomical."

"So?"

"Yeah, so. This is a disaster." Anders needed time to think. He circled the table. The obvious answer was that the children's embryos came from the same mother. Most patients produced more embryos than they used. Any leftovers, following a successful pregnancy, were stored in liquid nitrogen. Could they have found their way into all of these different patients? Doubtful. Redundant controls would prevent it.

His expression grew agitated. "What am I missing," he mumbled.

A knock on the door interrupted his concentration. It swung out to reveal Amy. She appeared contrite, but anxious.

"Sorry to interrupt, Doctor. Two men from the FBI are waiting in your office. They're very insistent."

The conflicting priorities rolled across Anders' face for several more seconds before he turned to Rudy. "I gotta go."

He had almost reached the door when Rudy asked, "Any word on the other thing, the virus or whatever, that we couldn't identify?"

So much to do, so much to say, Anders thought. When Rudy had first discovered children with matches from different families, his obsessive-compulsive nature had led him to run additional broad spectrum tests. He detected an RNA sequence that he could not identify and that seemed out of place.

"I don't know. Let the CDC doctors figure it out. That's why they're here."

~

Roxio's nightclub was legendary among the San Francisco twenty-somethings who trolled south of Market Street. Its pulsing electronic beat, its shifting colors, its flashing schools of saucy young fish all tantalized Anne Czajkowska. Whenever she wasn't scheduled in the lab at UCSF until late the next day, the thirty-three-year-old Polish biologist stalked Roxio's late-night crowd, a huntress of the dancing prey.

Tonight, Anne was bored. No one new or interesting sparked her desire. It wasn't early and it wasn't promising. Then it dawned on her that she was thinking about work. Outrageous. She couldn't have that. She shook her blond hair, stepped back from the edge of the dance floor, and eyed the bar. Her antenna piqued when she saw a striking Middle-Eastern man lead two men and a woman to a small table. The handsome man was about to sit when Anne saw him glance her way.

She saw him turn slowly to talk with the woman and was immediately attracted to her small bones, deep olive skin, and raven hair; her lips invited attention and her eyes challenged you to get it. Anne's skin prickled. Her stomach felt weak. That woman knew she could own the room. Unconsciously, Anne ran one hand through her short spiky hair.

The man turned away. Anne couldn't tell what he was saying, but she thought she saw the girl's eyes flick in her direction. A waitress arrived at their table, helped the group take their seats, and waited for their drink order. After a long pause, the waitress gazed around, bored, found Anne staring, and rolled her eyes.

Anne smiled back. Her insides churned in anticipation, but she would give the new arrivals time to settle before making her move. She stepped closer to the crowd and contemplated the dancers without seeing them behind the excitement and desire that enflamed her thoughts. How to begin?

A musky perfume caught her nostrils and instantly immersed her in a storybook palace in an ancient time, in a room of gold inlaid dark wood panels while she lay on giant velvet pillows. The image subsumed her so profoundly that she gasped and felt self-conscious. She turned left to look at the bar and was startled to see the olive-skinned woman standing very close. *Young*, Anne thought. Then, the girl's fragrance, the aroma of destiny, invaded her senses and she knew with certainty that the evening's promise would be fulfilled.

She turned to Anne and braved a small smile, indicating with a nod that she wanted to dance. Anne didn't hesitate. She smiled in return, put one arm around the girl's waist, and ushered her into the swaying crowd.

Just when they found room to move, the DJ slowed the tempo. The floor thinned out. The young girl smiled to show it was okay and Anne took the lead. She gently pressed her close and felt the heat pour from the girl's body as she rested her head on Anne's shoulder.

After a few minutes, Anne thought she heard a snuffle. She pulled back far enough to see the girl's face. Her skin was flushed. Her eyes flooded with tears. "What's this?" asked Anne, wondering whether the girl would mistake her Polish accent for a Russian one, like so many people did. A little game she played, a test of worldliness.

"It is just one of those, how you say, one of those days," the girl responded with a distinctive Italian cadence.

Anne squeezed her hand and thought for a moment. "Boyfriend?"

The girl nodded. Anne felt she had to lighten the mood and directed their steps through a flourish.

"Men," she added. "What do they know?"

The girl seemed troubled.

"He is ostetrico—"

"Obstetrician," Anne translated.

"Yes. He must know something about women."

"Only our cunts, my dear. Not the important parts."

The girl laughed and Anne squeezed her closer.

"I can soothe your ache, Little One. My apartment is just a few steps from here. You want to feel good?"

With the girl's head on her shoulder, Anne couldn't see the triumphant smile blossom to her lips.

~

Anders' eighth floor office overlooked the San Francisco Bay. If he put his nose on the floor-to-ceiling window and looked left he could see Alcatraz. The two FBI agents ferreting around the lavish suite hadn't discovered this yet. John Torsloff, the paternal, fifty-five-year-old member of the duo was more interested in the Asian collectables. The artfulness of the Chinese landscapes and delicate jades was wasted on Simon Keeler, the thirty-year-old button-down lawyer.

Keeler watched sailboats on the Bay. Torsloff hovered beside the enormous desk centered in the office and toyed with a small carved elephant.

"Ivory," Torsloff said, thinking about anti-poaching laws and customs restrictions. "Wonder when he got it."

The office door opened and Anders entered, removing his surgical cap as he crossed the room.

The agents, caught off guard, reached for their ID cards. Anders did not react to their sudden gestures.

"Doctor van der Veer, hello," Torsloff said as he replaced the elephant on Anders' desk. "Your receptionist said to wait here."

When Anders reached his desk, he glanced down first at Torsloff's ID and then at Keeler's. He remained standing. Determined to control the situation, height always gave him an advantage.

"We're really stacked up here, gentlemen. What can I do for you?"

Torsloff spoke first. "Your clinic seems to be the epicenter of an unexplained illness."

"Well, we've got a few children with flu-like symptoms. I didn't realize it had become a concern outside of our clinic."

Keeler stepped in.

"We got a call this morning from the Center for Disease Control in Atlanta."

"Yes, they've been investigating it for several days," Anders replied. "What's your interest?"

"This could be a national security issue," Keeler's voice was flat.

"Not sure I follow," said Anders.

"We're concerned with the origin of the disease," Keeler said, making it sound self-evident.

"We are too," snapped Anders. "Children, who began life in this clinic, are sick. We don't know the exact nature of the disease or the cause, but they are our children, in a sense, and we feel responsible to find an answer."

"What Agent Keeler means," said Torsloff, hoping to quell the sparring, "is that we're under the gun to determine whether the presence of this disease resulted from an action by a hostile agent. I'm sure you will acknowledge—"

Anders cut him off. "We're under a gun too," he said, his tone growing impatient. "We've got a much more pressing issue—"

"National security, Doctor."

Torsloff stayed Keeler with a gesture.

Anders rebooted. "Let me explain. One of our couples had a DNA paternity test come back negative. They believe there was a mix-up in our lab and the wife received someone else's embryos."

"Oops," Keeler touched his lips with his fingers.

"We don't make those kinds of mistakes, Agent Keeler."

The agent smirked.

"I can see why that concerns you," Torsloff's voice grew incredulous. "But is it more important than an illness from a potentially hostile source?"

"Definitely. Even the rumor of a mix-up could ruin us," Anders said. "It's already ruined the lives of our patients. Think of how the family with misplaced children feels."

"Betrayed, I would imagine," Torsloff said.

"Exactly. Our patients and their health come first. Our reputation, which depends on them, comes second. To us, the illness is a tertiary issue."

Keeler just shook his head. "When did you first learn there was an illness?"

"When our lab tech did the paternity test for the couple I mentioned he spotted an irregularity and made a routine call to the CDC to help identify it. Not a big deal."

"Well, it is officially a big deal," Torsloff said.

"Okay. We've got a few sick children and the CDC setting up camp here at the Hilton. And, as of today, you too. But I'm not so sure it's a big deal," Anders said.

"Please explain, Doctor," Torsloff shot back.

"Well, my gut tells me it's a virus. They'll run a few tests, figure it out, and then everyone will go home. If you want more information about the disease, I suggest you talk to the CDC. After that, if I can help, I will. But for now, you'll have to excuse me, but we've got a more troubling threat on our hands."

~

Anne lay on her back, her right arm behind her blond head and her left encircling the delicious dark-skinned creature that had entwined itself around her body. *One does not meet unshackled lust every day,* she thought. *What kind of torment lives in that perfect physique to radiate those gigawatts of emotion? And where did she get this flawless satiny hide?*

Her head spun. She could barely see candlelight flickering on the walls in her huge loft. But it showed the Rodin sculpture, solemn in its place at the edge of the broad carpet, that defined the loft's sleeping area. It stared at her like it knew she was disoriented. "What are you doing?" it seemed to ask. "Who is this woman?" Anne's mind was filled with passion and she dismissed the questions, lay back, and giggled to herself.

She felt a stir and when the girl glanced up at her, Anne looked back and smiled.

"I do not usually go to bed with someone I don't know their name," Anne whispered.

"Is—" her voice caught and she had to clear her throat. "Theresa." Anne felt the girl's body squeeze tighter and the word "insecure" popped to her mind.

"Well, Theresa, you didn't exactly take your time catching me."

"Only a little," she laughed and her eyes twinkled mischief.

"Were you worried I could escape?" Anne teased and then saw Theresa give a sly grin.

"Does mouse escape cat?"

Anne shifted onto her left arm, rolling Theresa off to her side. She gave her a mock serious face. "Depends. Which one is more hungry?"

"Me," Theresa said without hesitation. "I am more hungry."

"Me," Anne shook her head in slow disagreement. "I am still hungry." She growled and Dracula-lunged at Theresa's throat and forgot all of her questions.

~

Anders pulled open the door to his partner's office with purpose. His suite was identical to Anders' except for the furnishings: Anders liked Zen; Conrad was strictly Herman Miller.

Anders strode across the room to the standup desk where his fifty-year-old partner was working at a computer. Conrad Hughes had the bearing of an Army colonel, which he had been, and the vocabulary of a drill sergeant, which kept his subordinates, both in and out of the military, off-guard. Anders set his briefcase on the floor, snapped open the latch, and withdrew a sheet of paper.

As he straightened, he felt Conrad's eyes travel from the computer screen to his face.

"Anders," his tone was curt. "You solve this thing yet?"

Anders placed the paper on Conrad's desk and watched his partner grab it and scan. Anders waited until he'd finished before he spoke.

"I can't resolve this maternity issue."

Conrad stared back at him, silent and intense. *God, he can be an inscrutable bastard*, Anders thought.

"Jesus, Anders," the words came without force as if he couldn't believe it. He shook his head, turned aside, and let the paper drop onto the desk. Conrad strolled to the window, clasped his hands behind him, and stared at the San Francisco Bay.

"You told me this kind of thing was impossible."

Anders stepped to the window and stood beside Conrad who was tall, but just shy of Anders. They both gazed at the sailboats.

"It was," Anders replied, knowing what would come next.

"It isn't," he turned to Anders, his voice gaining momentum. "Two weeks. Four reports. Six children, all in different cities, all with the same DNA, and all from our clinic."

"I know," Anders turned to Conrad. "Rudy and I have been over the results. We agree that it's unimaginable. But it is what it is and we will find the cause."

"This is a colossal fuckup."

"In order for these children to have the same mitochondria DNA, they had to come from the same mother."

"So someone screwed up in the lab."

"Our controls are rigorous. They would normally prevent us from implanting the wrong embryos. It is a known risk and we designed procedures to avoid it. I'm not saying it's impossible, but I'm not ready to conclude someone screwed up."

Conrad retained the clarity and logic that had served him well in the military. It didn't surprise Anders that he went straight to the bottom line.

"Christ, Anders. We have patients in most states and half a dozen countries. Where's this thing going to stop?"

Conrad walked back to the desk, picked up the paper he'd dropped, and turned toward Anders. He waved it in front of him.

"How many maternity cases is this going to cause, at a million dollars each, in case you haven't read the papers lately? So much for our highly profitable business."

Anders knew the consequences, but he couldn't explain the cause. "I am positive it did not happen here. Whatever the origin, we'll get to the bottom of it."

Conrad surprised Anders. He dropped the paper and turned toward the door. Anders followed the look and realized that he had been so intent on meeting Conrad that he'd overlooked a man reading at a table by the entrance.

Conrad pointed to the man, who sat oblivious to their discussion. An American-Chinese, he looked to be in his forties and wore the outrageous hair and clothes of an Elvis impersonator.

"You didn't meet Richard Yi in Afghanistan, but he and I did some damage there when we served together. He's an ex-San Francisco cop, but he's still connected. He's here to help. Work with him. You need to wrap this up fast before our balls land in the duck fat."

Anders saw that the man still hadn't acknowledged that he'd heard them. Conrad raised his voice another notch.

"Richard. Would you take this fine young tiger with you to meet Sergeant Hong?"

Richard smiled. He rose casually to his feet and strolled toward them with a gait that reminded Anders of a duck waddling across his driveway. He eventually reached them and offered his hand. Anders took it. "Sergeant Hong?" he asked.

Richard spoke in a melodious baritone. The voice on top of the getup caused Anders to grin.

"He may have info on one of the techs working in your lab the day of the Davidson's procedure," Richard said. "We want to know if there was any possibility the tech could have mishandled the embryos whether by accident or on purpose."

"On purpose?" Anders asked. "Who would want to do that?"

"That's what we want to find out," Richard said. "I was just getting ready to boogie. Gotta meet him in thirty. How about it, Anders? You wanna join me?"

Anders thought his morning needed a break. He checked his watch. Conrad nodded. That settled it. The two men headed for the door, but Conrad stopped them with a Colombo-like question.

"Anders, could this have any connection to your enhanced fertilization procedure?"

Anders halted in mid-stride. The idea hadn't occurred to him.

"I can't see how, but I'll review it."

Conrad shrugged as if it was just a random thought and returned to his computer.

~

Anne held Theresa's hand while they crossed Green Street and headed up Grant. She liked walking the roundabout way to Washington Square. There were windows to shop, fantasies to explore, and Theresa had told her she hadn't visited this part of the city.

When they stopped to admire the clothes in an upscale boutique, Anne thought it was time to learn more about her new companion.

"So, this boyfriend," she began, reaching into Theresa's dark hair with her fingers and teasing her scalp.

"He owns a fertility clinic," Theresa replied. "I work in the lab."

"No." Anne frowned and let her hand fall to her side. "Not for a man who dumps you."

"Is okay." Theresa gave a little shrug. "I am smarter than him."

Anne smacked Theresa's behind. The girl's head whipped around and her eyes flashed. *Was it anger or uncertainty?* Anne wasn't sure.

"Oh." Anne arched an eyebrow and smiled. "Nice ass *and* a brain."

"Yes." An intriguing pout emerged on Theresa's lips. "Doctor of Microbiology, thank you, from Geneva."

"Really?" Anne felt the elation of coincidence. "I once knew a man there who taught polymerase chain reactions."

Now Theresa acted surprised.

"You know Israel Zudovich?"

"No." Anne turned wistful. "Only his name. His work led me to human reproductive cloning."

"Zudovich was good teacher to me. For him, I write algorithm to diagnose infectious disease."

What twist of the stars bought you into my life, Anne wondered. *You're perfect.*

"Then I study gene sequencing in Marseilles," Theresa continued.

"You really do know more than this boyfriend."

Theresa accepted the compliment, took Anne's hand, and led her up the sidewalk. Her voice softened with intimacy.

"But you? Cloning humans is not legal."

Anne glanced up at the clear sky hoping she wouldn't pursue the subject.

"Can be done?" the child insisted.

"Oh yes," Anne said, waving off any doubt. She felt Theresa turn to her and saw the question in her eyes.

"With mammals there are—so many die."

"That was true in the past," Anne said. "Today, I have 99 percent healthy reproduction while we are permitted to keep the embryos alive."

"Fourteen days is not a healthy baby."

Anne held Theresa eyes, not sure what to think. The girl knew California law and much more. "No, it is not," she said at last.

"How can you do this? It is difficult, no?"

"Yes and no," Ann looked at Theresa. "We start with somatic cell nuclear transfer. You know this, of course?"

"Yes. Where you remove nucleus from one egg and replace it with nucleus of egg taken from donor that you will clone."

"Exactly. But before we implant the donor nucleus, we use new reagents to purify the DNA and allow it to reproduce faithfully. Then, after the egg has received the donor nucleus, we have a process to facilitate methylation of the DNA. You know what that is?"

"When egg divides and cells become specialized, methylation tells genes in new cells to make more of the same kind. No need to remind liver cell to make more liver cells."

"See? You know everything."

"Not everything. But I know that if methylation is not correct, embryo will not develop healthy."

"Right again. The hard part is activating methylation so that the cells behave properly."

"You can do that?"

Ann smiled at her.

After a moment, Theresa's expression grew serious. "This would be good to know."

~

Anders couldn't remember ever riding in a Cadillac Seville and certainly not in one like this two-toned burgundy and silver behemoth. Though he had to admit that the pristine white interior communicated overindulgence in a manner his BMW never would.

Richard drove—very carefully—through the congested streets of North Beach. Anders found everything about him puzzling.

"This is some car."

"It's a 1977. Last model The King owned. I'd ride you in my Stutz Blackhawk, but I don't drive it in the city. Wherever I parked, it'd be gone in sixty seconds."

Richard stopped to let pedestrians cross. When he started up, Anders caught his look.

"Conrad says you were in the Dutch Army."

"I was a medical officer assigned to the Korps Comandotroepen," Anders corrected him.

"That's the special operations group, right?

"The KTC is equivalent to your Green Berets. We wore green berets."

"But you were a doc so they let you off easy in training, right?"

Anders smiled. "No. We all went through the same torture. Only 30 percent of those who start finish with the beret."

"Well, you must have done okay," Richard said. "Conrad said you were his best trauma doc in The Stan."

"Yeah?" Anders turned away and contemplated his response. "There was a bloody fight in Nuristan, near the Paki border, and Conrad requested head trauma specialists. The Dutch were south, in Uruzgan, but I volunteered. Their injuries were quite grim, but we managed to save several difficult cases. Somehow, Conrad got my commandant to second me to his staff and I stayed with him through the rest of my tour."

"I remember it," Richard said. "I was in Army intelligence. I helped him investigate the battle. Afterwards, I started doing his intelligence work." He paused. "Did you see any fighting?"

Anders hated the question. "Unfortunately, we did. It was precarious for many months."

"Conrad also said the fertility clinic was your idea."

"It was. We became friends. I had an idea to help families who wanted children. I liked obstetrics in med school. As a lawyer, Conrad knew how to run a business. He thought the idea had potential so we teamed up."

"And now you have a situation." Richard took his eyes from the road and stared at Anders for what he thought was a dangerously long time. Finally, he asked, "So tell me how patients get the wrong embryos."

"Know anything about IVF?"

"My wife does." Richard leaned back and smiled. "She thinks in vitro fertilization is a crime against nature."

Anders decided to pass on the wife's comment.

"We inject the woman with hormones so she will produce a dozen or more eggs."

"The wife hates shots." Richard grimaced.

"Each patient has a color code for her charts," Anders continued. "Lab dishes, partner's sperm collection material— everything. We count the oocytes, the eggs, and store them in incubators."

"Can someone open an incubator without anyone knowing?"

"Uh-uh," Anders replied. "Open a door, you set off alarms. A precaution to stabilize the temperature, keep the eggs healthy."

The car slowed and stopped beside an empty parking space, a rarity in this part of town. Anders admired Richard's perfect parallel parking. Richard killed the ignition and turned to Anders with a deadpan expression. "Did you know Elvis was a Jew?"

Anders wasn't sure he heard right.

"What?"

"I just found out," Richard said, with deep concern. "I'm thinking of converting."

His face was so serious, Anders could not think of a suitable reply. He reached for the door handle.

Out on Green Street, Anders found himself half a step behind Richard heading toward a four-story warehouse. Surprised at the shorter man's brisk pace he stretched his own legs until he came beside him.

"As I was saying," Anders continued the explanation. "The man donates his sperm—"

"Ha." Richard cut him off with a staccato laugh. "A guy I knew underwent the procedure. Said afterwards, whenever he walked down the Tupperware isle at the market, he got a hard-on."

Anders laughed. An enigma, but not dull.

"We mix the sperm and eggs, culture the embryos for a couple of days until they're ready to go back into the patient."

"All of them?" Richard asked.

"No, one or two. Used to be more. But I developed a procedure that gives us a pregnancy with every healthy embryo."

"What about leftovers?" In spite of his banter, Richard noted details.

"We store them in liquid nitrogen in case the patient wants more children later."

Anders followed Richard through the lobby of a building and into a carpeted hallway that smelled like burnt toast. They entered the stairwell and walked to the second floor where the light was brighter and the smell disappeared.

"Can anyone get into the lab alone?" Richard asked over his shoulder. He walked down the hall reading suite numbers.

"Normally, it's locked," Anders said from behind. "There are always two people inside when it's open."

Richard stopped before an apartment door and regarded Anders over one shoulder.

"Okay. I now understand IVF," he paused. "But I'll ask again: How did your patients' embryos get mixed up?"

"That's why you're here," Anders said with a smile.

Richard held Anders' eyes, but reached with one fist and knocked on the door. Anders saw that he didn't wait for an answer before pushing it open.

He followed Richard into an empty loft that must have belonged to an artist. Twelve foot ceilings over forty-by-seventy feet of polished hardwood floors and windows the entire length of one wall.

At the far end, a policeman stood next to the window resting one boot on the sill and balancing a slim folder on his upraised knee. His uniform was trim and he appeared to be in his late twenties.

"Jerry, all's well?" Richard said as they strode across the shiny floor. Anders wondered at the stark emptiness of the apartment.

Sergeant Jerry Hong exhaled a lungful of cigarette smoke before he replied.

"Well? Yeah, if I overlook my wife's bitching 'cause we're not going to Hawaii for Christmas."

"Wonderful," Richard said. "Who told you to marry a Hawaiian?" The men stopped before the policeman. Hong looked down at the folder, opened it, and cradled it in the crook of his arm. With his free hand he brought the cigarette to his mouth.

"I'd say it's nice to see you too, Inspector Yi but I know you like to get right to the point. So, what do you guys want to know?"

"It's just Richard, these days, Jerry. No longer Inspector. Tell us about the lab assistant."

"I remember talking to the roommate," Hong replied. "We got a missing persons report." He glanced at a sheet inside the folder.

"This roommate was a thirty-two-year-old Caucasian woman. In the US, uh, overstayed her visa, actually. Said she woke up Sunday morning, October 7th, and the girl wasn't there. Nothing missing."

Anders felt nauseous. His heart pounded. He was dizzy and

needed to sit. He shuffled to the nearest window.

"October a year ago?" he asked as he landed abruptly on the sill.

Hong didn't raise his head, just nodded, and continued to read.

"The roommate said she was worried. Apparently, this girl was the adventuresome type."

"Yeah?" Richard raised his eyebrows.

"So," Hong continued. "I took down the details, poked around, saw nothing amiss, and filed the paperwork. Didn't hear anything about it until July."

Despite his discomfort, Anders knew he must give his full attention.

"The Coast Guard recovered a woman's body off Baker Beach. Same age, description as this assistant, Theresa Lanzatella. According to the Coroner, she died around the same time Theresa disappeared."

In spite of himself, the news shocked Anders. Theresa had left after a terrible fight. He'd heard nothing from her for the last year. Now she was dead! The deep longing he'd felt in his gut for the past year suddenly threatened to take over his body.

"Anything to positively identify this body?" he heard Richard ask.

"No. But he thinks it was her. Physical similarity. Timing. It's pretty strong. Theresa was the only woman reported missing at the time the corpse drowned."

"Drowned?" Anders didn't know whether he sounded casual.

The sergeant studied the paper again and read.

"Death by asphyxia due to submersion, with aspiration of salt water."

"No dental records?" Richard asked. Anders thought Richard was studying him even though he directed his question to Hong. He hid his sadness and hoped the former policeman couldn't see.

"Nope," said Hong and stubbed his cigarette out on a piece of scrap wood lying on the sill.

Anders sensed that Richard's gaze lingered before he turned

again to the sergeant.

"How do we find this roommate?"

"She worked at UCSF on Parnassus. I got the number here—" Hong held up the only sheet of paper in the folder and flipped it over. "Somewhere."

This time, Anders felt Richard's dark eyes look right through him.

"So, Doc," asked the recondite Elvis. "Where's this leave us?"

Anders felt like he walked into a door. Worse, he was trapped. He sat on the window ledge and looked back at Richard. He knew he couldn't hide his feelings, but now wasn't the time to explain. After a moment, he stood and shrugged like he didn't know or couldn't say.

~

Anne rejoiced when she saw no waiting line at Mama's Cafe. She didn't know the waitress who ushered them into the bubble-gum-pink room, but at least they had a table. They gave their order and Anne watched the waitress head to the kitchen before placing both forearms on the table, palms up, inviting Theresa to hold her hands.

"So, when did you come into The Life?" Anne's voice sounded offhand.

"Is difficult." The girl placed her hands in Anne's and lowered her eyes.

"Just a hint, then."

Theresa seemed to consider for a moment then raised her head and caught Anne with a chilling look, a granite face, and sharp grey eyes that drilled into her soul. Anne shivered.

"Mama's boyfriend," Theresa's voice was hollow. "He hurt me bad. I was ten. After, Mama's brothers take him away."

"I'm sorry." Anne felt a prickle of sweat on her back.

"Yes. But now I get even." The malevolent eyes grew darker for a moment and then lightened just as quickly. Anne saw again the pleasant girl who'd been her companion since last night, her eyes now moist with compassion.

"How about you? You will marry? Have baby someday?"

The change was so sudden. Anne, caught off guard, felt the first sting of tears. She looked down at their hands.

"I don't think so," she murmured. "Not possible. Not yet."

She pulled one hand away and reached into her blazer pocket for a tissue.

"Ah. Is why you study cloning?" Said like a discovery, but intended to console. Anne wanted to hide. It wasn't difficult.

"Humanity needs a plan," her voice grew intense. "Cloning is the next logical step in assisted reproduction and we must stop viewing it as a transgression of nature. Look at the benefits. Infertile couples could have a genetically related child. So could same sex couples. They could avoid transmitting undesirable genes. Parents who lost a child could find comfort in a genetic copy. Besides all of that, it gives us a way to better ourselves. Improve our best traits."

Theresa's face showed no emotion. "One day you will make full-baby clones?"

Anne retrieved her other hand from the table, blew her nose, and then regarded Theresa for a long time before she answered.

"Yes. I will."

Theresa glanced furtively at the other diners and then conspiratorially at Anne.

"I know you will."

~

Anders knew Conrad wanted to see him but the meeting with Sergeant Hong had distracted him. As he hurried through the corridor to his partner's office, he felt a sudden anxiety. *Had he forget his notes? Damn.* He stopped and riffled the contents of the clipboard in his hand.

He found the notes and, at the same time, heard footsteps behind him. He saw the two FBI agents approaching and did not contain his displeasure.

"You're back," he said without smiling.

"Yup," said Torsloff. Keeler just nodded with a smirk. More footsteps, this time from the hallway ahead, caused them all to turn toward the sound. Conrad and Richard come bustling around a corner, but stopped dead at the sight of the three men.

"Anders," Conrad blurted. "We need you."

"On my way," he turned to the agents. "Gentlemen, this is my partner, Conrad Hughes." He turned to Conrad. "These men are with the FBI."

"Good grief," Conrad was about to shake hands but let his drop. "Could this thing get any more complicated?"

Anders turned to Richard, "And this is—"

Both agents nodded to Richard, who nodded back.

"You all know each other?" Conrad observed. "Fine. In that case, C'mon, we're meeting the CDC in their temporary lab. Bastards are driving me nuts. Maybe we'll get some answers today."

Conrad headed down the corridor, leaving the others to follow.

The temporary lab was a storeroom that Conrad had made available to the CDC for analyses work. It was just big enough for a half a dozen people to squeeze shoulder-to-shoulder around a lab bench in the center of the floor.

Anders followed Conrad into the crowded space. The two agents and Richard brought up the rear. The three people standing around the cluttered bench stopped their animated discussion when they saw Conrad.

"Hello everyone," Conrad said. "You know my partner, Doctor van der Veer and you know these two gentlemen from the secret government bureaucracy. This is our security consultant, Richard Yi."

The newcomers nodded to the scientists and Conrad motioned to each one in turn.

"This is Doctor Benjamin Glick, communicable diseases. Doctor Arthur Li is a geneticist. Doctor Margaret Thierre is a molecular pathologist."

Anders had met the CDC officials when they first arrived, but had not learned their background. Glick appeared to be about sixty. He was probably the leader. Thierre was attractive and thirtyish with intelligent eyes. It was hard to figure out Li, who was no spring chicken and who immediately zeroed in on Richard. When he spoke, his accent was so stereotyped Anders almost laughed.

"You funny looking. Where you go to school?"

Anders watched Richard's eyes widen, hadn't thought it possible for anyone to disturb his *wa*.

"Cal Poly," Richard said, somewhat astonished. Then, "You don't look so hot yourself."

"Me, Peking University. PhD, Duke."

Conrad didn't waste time with pissing contests. He moved between them. "Glad you're getting on fellas, but we got business."

Glick took the cue and addressed Anders.

"Doctor van der Veer, we have finally made some progress with your disease."

"Good. What have you got?"

"The gene sequence your technician discovered resembles an Arboviral Encephalitides found in Asia," Glick said.

"Virus confirmed." Anders cast a knowing smile at the two FBI agents and then nodded with approval to Glick. "What do you know about it?"

Glick turned to Li, who hurried around the table and stopped beside Anders with a toothy smile.

"I explain for everyone," Li said. Anders felt him touch his right wrist with one finger. "Virus enter blood stream from bite of infected insect." He continued to smile and reached up to touch Anders forehead. "Localize in the brain, inflame tissue, and surrounding membrane." Li illustrated each statement with a forceful gesture.

"White blood cells rush to site. Fight infection," his comical voice escalated. "Create more swelling. Bleeding in the brain. Dead nerve cells. Brain damage. Maybe death."

Anders felt Conrad shudder beside him. "This is what those sick children downstairs can expect?"

At that moment, Keeler stepped to one side for a better view of Glick and drew Anders attention. He scrutinized the FBI agent while Glick spoke.

"Your virus is from Saudi Arabia. It's a flavivirus, related to one from the southern Indian state of Karnataka, home of Bangalore, and to another from Omsk in Siberia. Their fatality is about 30 percent."

Keeler glanced at Torsloff and mouthed the words "Saudi Arabia."

Anders turned to Glick. "Not very encouraging."

"What the hell's a flavivirus?" Conrad interrupted.

"Mr. Hughes," Glick looked at Conrad. "It's part of a family of viruses called Flaviviridae that spread mainly through ticks and mosquitoes. Flavivirus is a genus of that family. It includes Yellow Fever, Dengue fever, West Nile Virus, and others that may cause encephalitis. These viruses are simple and very clever. They have an RNA genome and replicate in the cytoplasm of the host cells."

"Whoa. You need to explain that for me," Conrad said. "I'm a lawyer, remember?" He waved his hand for Glick to continue.

"Doctor, if I may," the French microbiologist stepped forward. Glick motioned for her to proceed.

Thierre pick up a marker pen and drew a large diagram of a cell on the table. She added details to the drawing as she explained viral replication in melodic, accented English.

"In this cell, we have a small nucleus here at the center, floating in a lot of cytoplasm and all contained within a membrane.

"Along comes a virus. It wants to reproduce but some of the material it needs exists only in the host, which is why viruses can replicate only from inside a living cell. Viruses are designed to invade a host cell, reprogram it to make more viruses instead of more host cells, and lastly, send the new viruses to infect other hosts."

She paused and looked at Conrad. "You know what are DNA and RNA?"

Conrad nodded. "I've heard of them, yes."

Thierre missed the sarcasm in Conrad's tone and continued. "In cells, DNA is responsible for inheritance and RNA for synthesizing proteins. I will explain some of the process so you will understand what is happening with your patients. Okay?"

Conrad nodded, yes.

She sketched a double-helix beside her illustration of a cell. "You've seen this drawing of DNA, yes? Deoxyribonucleic acid. Most people interpret it as a spiral staircase. The two strands of the double helix are identical, but joined head to tail, in opposite directions. We need to understand the structure of only one of the helixes. It consists of a chain of molecular units called nucleotides. A nucleotide has three chemical components: a sugar, a phosphate, and a nitrogenous base. Sugar and phosphate molecules align alternately to form the spiral strand of the helix. One of the nitrogenous bases—either adenine, cytosine, guanine, or thymine —attaches at a right angle to a sugar on the strand. This bond completes the nucleotide and forms one step in the staircase. Other steps, other nucleotides, may contain any of the four bases."

Conrad guffawed. "Will there be a test?"

"No," Thierre smiled and tapped the drawing with the marking pen.

"Just remember this: the sequence of nucleotides, the steps along one strand of the staircase, determines the sequence of the amino acids in a particular protein."

"Well, that much I can remember," Conrad smiled at Thierre. "But what does it mean for our patients?"

"We're getting to that," Thierre gave Conrad a sympathetic glance. "Let me continue. I will leave out some of the chemistry so it is not difficult."

Conrad turned his palms up to acknowledge that she should continue.

"Here is RNA," she said and drew a single helix beside the double helix. "It looks like DNA split lengthwise. The RNA molecule in combination with different enzymes performs protein synthesis in three stages and for each stage we give it a different name. For the first stage, enzymes in the cell nucleus unwind the

DNA helix and copy the nucleotide sequence of one strand to make a molecule called messenger RNA. You see?" She drew a long string with many small spikes protruding from one side. "Each spike represents one nucleotide."

"Okay," Conrad acknowledged.

"The messenger RNA leaves the nucleus and enters the cytoplasm where it finds a healthy supply of amino acids. Now a second molecule, ribosomal RNA, which is shaped more like a glob than a string, wraps around one end of the messenger RNA strand. It identifies the first nucleotide on the string and waits for a third molecule, transfer RNA, to bring it the corresponding amino acid. It grabs the acid, moves to the next nucleotide on the messenger string, and, when the transfer RNA delivers the second corresponding amino acid, links them together. It repeats this procedure, assembling a complete protein by the time it reaches the end of the messenger RNA strand."

She looked again to see whether Conrad understood.

"I'm with you so far," Conrad said.

"Good," Thierre said. "Now we return to the virus. It has arrived at the host. It contains either DNA or RNA but not both. Each type must reproduce along a separate path. A virus with DNA must make messenger RNA before it can make proteins. It carries its genetic code into the host's nucleus. As part of the host's normal cycle, it replicates the virus along with its own DNA.

"Whereas, other viruses, like the Alkhurma virus, contain messenger RNA. They forego a trip to the nucleus and stop in the cytoplasm where they start immediately to use the host's ribosomes and amino acids to make proteins.

"With both evolutions, the result is the same: the virus directs the cell to make proteins for a new virus. These proteins assemble into a virus, which then breaks out of the host cell and often kills it in the process."

"Damn," said Conrad.

No one spoke. The CDC doctors waited while the clinic administrators absorbed the information. Finally Dr. Li broke the silence.

"We have many genome sequences of Arborvirus in our database," Li said. "We compare sequence in your patients to our database, we got 89 percent match to Alkhurma Hemorrhagic Fever Virus from Saudi Arabia."

"Good," said Anders hoping that a positive ID would mean progress.

Li gave a sharp bark that was intended as a laugh.

"Except for parts don't match."

"Not good?"

Anders saw the French microbiologist turn toward him. "Doctor van der Veer, the virus has been modified. It will be more aggressive."

"Modified how?" Torsloff jumped in.

"We believe that a sequence of nucleotides was added to the viral RNA," Thierre said. "It enables the formation of a protein, a catalyst to speed up replication. Your virus multiplies faster than the original Alkhurma virus. It will be more lethal."

"Not good again," Anders mused. "Prognosis?"

"Probably fatal to anyone who is infected now," Anders caught her expression of sympathy. "However, you recall that a virus reproduces by a different path whether it contains DNA or RNA?"

"Yes," Anders said.

"DNA viruses are stable because an enzyme called DNA polymerase corrects mistakes in new copies of DNA molecules during replication. That is why vaccines for DNA viruses remain effective for years. But RNA polymerase is less effective at reducing errors during RNA replication. This means that your Alkhurma virus will mutate with each generation and eventually grow benign."

"But not before it does a lot of damage," Anders said.

"Hey!" Conrad interjected. "We got a ward with sick kids. How are we going to cure them?"

"Difficult, Mister Hughes," Thierre said. "We can see the result of the altered RNA virus, but we need to identify the sequence of nucleotides that is responsible in order to disrupt it."

Anders saw Torsloff lean forward again.

"How'd the virus travel from Saudi Arabia?" the agent asked.

"We do not know yet." Thierre shrugged.

"What's more important," said Conrad, "is how do we stop it?"

Anders saw Torsloff motion Keeler toward the door.

"Gentlemen and lady," Torsloff said. "It's been great. You've obviously got important work to do. We'll leave you to it." Then he turned to Anders. "Doctor, we'll be in touch."

~

The morning sunshine and the blue sky soothed Anne's spirits. She lifted her face to the warmth as she guided Theresa across Filbert Street and into Washington Square Park. Breakfast had been good. The girl had impressive knowledge of her work. What a find.

She felt Theresa take her arm and draw it tight to her body.

"What if I take your clones and trade them for embryos in the clinic."

"You can't be serious." Anne peered at her in astonishment.

"Yes," her voice rose with childish enthusiasm. "It is perfect idea. Many women can have your babies."

Anne drew the idea into focus: preposterous, but not impossible. Competitors already claimed success birthing cloned embryos in Russia and the Middle East where the prospect of advancing science outweighed the stigma of creating an ungodly child. Suddenly, she smelled coffee. Theresa leaned her head close to whisper.

"No one would know. Mothers would love babies."

It was absurd. Of course someone would know.

"They would find out," Anne shook her head.

"Is it not your dream?" the girl's eyes were searching her face. "To give women the better way to have children?"

Yes, it was her selfish dream. Just because she could not conceive in the traditional way, society shouldn't exclude her from having genetic offspring. She knew it was possible. She had already verified the initial steps. But the girl's vision didn't match her fantasy of announcing the breakthrough to the scientific community and relishing its accolades.

"Not like that," she said at last.

"No one else can do it," Theresa insisted. "Only you and me. We are the perfect team. You prove is possible. I make it happen. After, no one can deny it works."

Could it really be that simple? Anne wondered. *Swap a few embryos in the clinic and let them come to life in unsuspecting mothers? Pray to God there are no abnormalities. No,* she shook her head at the thought, *the mothers would eventually learn the truth.*

"But my DNA," Anne said. "They would know it was me."

"What about me?" Theresa asked.

"You? What are you thinking?" The girl was relentless. She didn't understand the long odds for success or its consequences.

"I have eggs," said Theresa. "Anders keep them for me in case I will wait before I make children."

"Frozen?"

"At the clinic. We could use them. You could teach me to clone embryos."

Anne could feel the brickwork guarding her confidence crumble as Theresa hammered her objections one by one. Still, no. What she proposed was no solution.

"Even if it worked," Anne said. "They will know your identity whenever someone tests their DNA."

"Fine," the girl replied with bravado. "The perfect insult. Anders, he dump me. I make him put my clones in his patients."

At last, light falls on the truth, Anne thought. She put an arm on Theresa's shoulder. They walked a few paces and then Anne squeezed the girl closer.

"You really hate the man."

Theresa lowered her face and concentrated on the ground a few steps ahead. When she raised her gaze, Anne saw for the second time the cold and penetrating eyes that had stunned her in the restaurant.

"We were lovers," Theresa said at last. "I wanted him to leave his wife. He said no. I had his baby inside me. He lie to me. He drug me and kill his baby. You can only hate such a man."

Anne felt her jaw drop. *Poor girl.* What kind of man, let alone a doctor, would do such a thing? An insensitive bastard; no, a callous criminal. An evil man who needed to learn a lesson. She glanced at Theresa. *One that she and I have the special skills to teach.*

Suddenly the pieces fell together and she knew. This girl had sought her out because she needed help to unleash her revenge on the doctor and his clinic. Theresa had blinded her with soft voluptuous beauty and passionate sex and convinced her to collaborate in an ethical crime that would change history.

"You know the bird that lays its eggs in nest of other bird?" The mischief returned to Theresa's eyes. "Is magpie, no?"

"A cuckoo," Anne corrected.

"I prefer magpie."

Pilgrim

Anders counted the occupied beds in the sick ward and realized he had eight new patients since his last visit. Suddenly, he feared that the arborvirus could be a more urgent threat than the misplaced embryos.

The CDC doctors had asked to join him on rounds so they could better understand his patients' condition. Conrad had accompanied them. They had just finished their last exam when Anders heard a mobile ring. He saw Conrad step away to take the call and Glick approach him with a troubled expression.

"Fever, vomiting, headache, swollen lymph glands," Glick said.

Anders knew what he was thinking.

"Quarantine," Anders said and then realized his mistake. "But there's no vector."

"You are correct," Thierre interjected. "The Alkhurma is an arborvirus, which means it is transmitted by the bite of an arthropod, tick, or mosquito. There are no ticks or mosquitoes here to carry the virus to a new host. However, the Alkhurma virus in these patients was engineered to find its way into the respiratory system. It becomes airborne."

Anders hadn't considered this.

"So anyone who comes in contact—"

"Precisely," replied the pathologist.

"It will spread fast," Anders acknowledged.

"Unfortunately," added Glick.

Anders thought of his patients. "Some of the effected families still have not brought their children in for observation," he said. "But the Davidson twins are on their way now. One shows signs of a clonic seizure."

Conrad had finished his call and now walked toward him pocketing the mobile. He questioned Anders with his eyes.

"Uncontrolled jerking movements," Anders explained to his partner. "Maybe onset of a seizure."

"Your patients are symptomatic of encephalitis in the first stage," Glick added turning to Conrad. "They're starting to enter the lethal second stage and—" he turned back to Anders. "Well, I don't have to tell you."

"How do we stop this damn virus?" With each word, Conrad's fists pounded the air in frustration.

"We stop it, Mr. Hughes, by silencing the genes that make the proteins necessary for the dangerous traits to replicate," Glick said. "If we succeed, it will lose those genes in future generations as well."

"Why didn't I think of that?" Conrad's sarcasm was cold.

"Let me explain," Glick backtracked. "Only certain sequences of the viral RNA gene are enabling it to replicate faster and reach the respiratory system. To the host cells, we can add a short strand of RNA with a code that is complementary to the harmful sequence in the native RNA. It will destroy all genes that carry the harmful sequence and stop production of their proteins."

"What's stopping us?" Conrad asked.

"We don't have the code sequence of the RNA so we cannot create a complementary one."

"Let's get on it," Conrad said. "While we're at it, explain to me whey we can't use your technique to shut down the whole damn thing? A complementary virus?"

"That's a good question, Mr. Hughes," Glick said. "It is another possible solution we are considering but it is a bit more involved. Meanwhile, we are running out of time."

Anders didn't know where to begin. He started for the door. The others followed.

Glick wasn't finished. "A delicate question, Doctor, but do you have frozen embryos leftover from the patients who now have sick children? Sibling embryos?"

"You're entering dangerous waters, even for the CDC," said Conrad, ever the attorney.

"National Security, Mister Hughes. I can certainly request a subpoena," Glick's request surprised Anders.

"But you already have swabs from the children," Anders began. Then he stopped with a flash of insight. Everyone stopped.

"Ah, but the embryos may have the original RNA virus," Anders said.

Li saw that Anders understood. "In children, virus mutate. We study original, maybe find sequence to prevent replication of bad properties. Save lives."

Anders turned to Li. "I'll see that you get what you need."

"Thank you," said Li. "Still, may need original schema. Map of data from person who make changes: notes, computer files. But now, we do our best with embryos."

Anders took another two steps toward the door then stopped again. His eyes lit up and he turned suddenly to Glick.

"What you just said about the second stage. It gives me an idea for the Davidson children."

Anders didn't wait for a response, but continued out the door into the corridor and disappeared.

Moments later, Anders arrived in the reception lobby. The Davidsons had just come through the door, each one clutching a child wrapped up like a papoose. Both babies sneezed and coughed and writhed in their parents arms.

"Good," he greeted them. "I'm glad you made it. This way, please." He ushered them to the elevator.

"They're really sick, Doctor," Rose had tears in her eyes. "What are you going to do?"

"We need your help," James said, his concern mirroring his wife's. "Do you know what's wrong yet?"

Anders gave them a solemn nod. Once they were all inside, he said, "As I explained on the phone, several children have matching symptoms, but we're still analyzing their condition and haven't found a cure yet."

The Davidsons exchanged looks of dismay.

"Not to worry. We're going to the ward. I've got a plan." Rose was too wrought to reply. James implored him with sad eyes.

The elevator doors opened, they stepped into the Sick Ward and two nurses took the twins from the Davidsons. Anders stepped ahead and barked an order to the charge nurse.

"Emily, get me five milligrams each of ketamine, amantadine, and midazolam. Send someone out if necessary."

"Right away," Amy hurried away, leaving Anders and the Davidsons to follow the two nurses to the far end of the ward where they made the twins comfortable in adjoining beds.

Rose and James knelt beside one of the beds. Anders walked to the opposite side, leaned over, and stroked the child's hair. He regarded the Davidsons.

"The body's immune system reacts so vigorously to attack from some viruses that it damages the brain. The defense kills the patient, not the virus. Rabies is like that."

"But there's no cure for rabies," Rose was horrified.

"Not exactly," Anders said.

"I heard that when you're bitten," Rose continued, "you get twenty-two shots in the stomach to keep from getting it. But once you've got it, you're dead, right?"

Anders gave both parents his most understanding smile.

"In 2004, a girl in Wisconsin was the first person we know of to survive rabies. A local doctor gave her sedatives and anti-inflammatories to protect her brain while the virus ran its course."

"She lived?" Rose couldn't believe it.

"Took a year," said Anders. "But she's well now."

Anders saw the three CDC doctors enter the ward and walk toward him between the double rows of beds. He decided to wait until he heard them out. Maybe they had more information. When they reached the twins' beds he introduced his patients.

"Doctors. Mister and Missus Davidson." Anders pointed to the twins who still writhed in their beds.

"These children are their twins. We were just discussing treatment." Before Anders could continue, Rose stood and looked Glick straight in the eye.

"Why can't you experts find a cure?" Contempt laced her tone, but Glick had seen her kind before.

"Missus—Davidson is it? It's rather a tricky problem. We identified the virus. We still need a way to treat children like yours that are already infected and, of course, keep it from spreading."

He should run for president, Anders thought.

"And?" Rose matched Glick's haughtiness.

"We're looking for the proverbial needle in a haystack," Glick explained. "A one-inch section of a string that reaches around the earth."

"So what do you think about Doctor van der Veer's treatment?" Rose continued. "Ketamine and some other stuff that has to do with rabies."

Anders caught Glick give him a look of censure.

"You're not thinking of the Milwaukee Protocol, are you?"

The rebuke surprised Anders, but he hid his displeasure. "I am," he said with confidence.

"The CDC has not had great success with Doctor Willoughby's method." Glick said.

Who is this guy to give me a lecture? Anders thought and felt heat surge to his temples. "That was rabies," he said quickly. "Besides, they didn't follow the protocol."

"What? An experiment? On my children?" Rose was not ready to hear details. Anders hoped he wasn't losing her.

"Rose, there's an excellent chance. The virus is similar to rabies —"

Glick interrupted. "Actually, it's closer to Yellow Fever. We have immunizations for that."

"At least in its progression," Anders continued, feeling himself on the defensive. "We want to prevent the immune system from killing the patient, like Willoughby did."

"By inducing a coma."

It sounded to Anders like Glick had chosen a path, could not turn back, and, instead, was going to badger them with sarcasm.

"Sweet Jesus!" Rose threw her hands above her head.

Anders grabbed Glick's upper arm and shoved him away from the group. He didn't care what the others thought. In his mind, Glick had already overstepped the bounds of professionalism. Anders stopped a dozen feet away, forced Glick around so they stood nose to nose, and snarled in a voice he could barely control.

"What are you doing?"

"I—I—was—" Glick obviously wasn't used to this kind of treatment.

"I'm trying to give these people some hope," Anders hissed. "Their children may die. The others, too."

"But it hasn't worked," Glick stammered.

"But it could work," Anders growled. "At least it's something. You've been here, what, three days? What have you done?"

"Doctor, that's unfair."

"*Doctor*, these are my patients. Stay out of it." Anders gave Glick's arm a determined squeeze, he hoped a painful one, and then released it with a snap of his wrist. From over his shoulder he heard Rose.

"What about my children?" she pleaded.

"We're just discussing them," Anders said, calming himself.

"It's okay, Missus Davidson," said Glick. "I believe Doctor van der Veer's plan is a good one." Then he glared at Anders. "Your best case here will be a temporary fix. We need a permanent cure. Don't you understand? We're running out of time. We need the original schema to stop this virus."

Anders knew Glick spoke the truth, but he had not completely recovered his temper.

"I will get it, *Doctor!*"

~

"This is your fault," Pryia again. It couldn't get any worse. Anders stared out the passenger-side window of Conrad's Acura at the wisps of fog racing in from the Pacific. How had he ever let things get so far beyond his control? His life was falling apart because of one mistake. No, it was more than one. Shame overwhelmed him. The cold feeling of Conrad's disappointment rolled over him from the driver's seat like the afternoon fog.

"What the bloody hell were you thinking?" Conrad boomed.

Anders saw scorn in his partner's sideways glance.

"It just happened, right?" The warm tone of Richard's baritone floating from the back seat emphasized the chill of his sarcasm. Anders felt his face grow taught. He stared up at the gray headliner. No escape. He had to tell them everything—well, not everything. Not how the blood surged in his groin when he first saw her. Not how her perfume destroyed his will power. Not how addicted he became to being in her presence.

"She was in my seminar at UCSF two summers ago. A brilliant student. She invited me to coffee."

"And you accepted with your prick?" Conrad shot back.

You couldn't stop Conrad when he got on a roll.

"She put me on to the new fertilization procedure."

"I thought that was your idea." Conrad said with surprise.

"It was. Just something she said during a procedure made me see the solution."

Conrad pulled to the curb and stopped the car. No one moved to get out. Richard leaned forward between the two front seats to see Anders' face.

"Anyway, you hired her." Richard urged him to continue.

"She said she wanted experience in a fertility clinic."

"Doing what?" Conrad taunted. "Collecting sperm by mouth?"

It wasn't like that, Anders thought. *Why can't I get this across? I'm not a total idiot.* "She was the best lab technician I ever saw. Best we ever had."

"Wait a minute," Conrad had warmed up. "Not the same girl who dropped the Petri dish and invoked the wrath of the Davidsons."

"Could happen to anyone." Conrad's eyes told Anders he thought it was bullshit.

"Then what?" Richard asked.

Anders dreaded this part. "She got pregnant," he said. "There were complications."

"Jesus," Conrad's head rolled back. "This gets better and better."

"No, it doesn't," Anders was outwardly calm. "She claimed I aborted the child without her consent. She said I did it save my marriage. Then she called Pryia and told her everything."

"Well, that explains your wife's little holiday," Conrad quipped.

Anders watched his partner reach for the door handle.

"I need food," Conrad said and pushed open the car door. Anders stepped out his side onto the sidewalk and towered above Richard as they waited for Conrad to come around the car.

When Conrad stepped over the curb Richard spoke in a somber voice. "Anders was screwing Theresa, but she also had a girlfriend."

"Christ!" said Conrad as he joined them to make a tight circle.

Richard removed a notepad from his jacket. He riffled through it and Anders felt humiliation warming his ears.

"Anne chaz-a-KOW-ski," Richard's voice made it sound like the title of a movie. "Know her?"

Anders was about to say, no, but caught himself.

"Wait. I do. Say it, chai-KOF-ski, like the composer. She's a geneticist. On the bleeding edge of reproductive cloning. What was she doing in San Francisco?"

"What the hell was she doing with our lab tech?" Conrad growled.

Anders saw Richard's baffled expression. Neither of them could answer.

"Anders, what's our exposure?" Conrad asked.

Good question, Anders thought. We have one of the world's experts on human cloning in an intimate relationship with my top lab tech. Cloning would explain the children with identical DNA profiles—but was it even possible?

He turned to Conrad. "With Czajkowska? Hard to say. Genetically altered embryos?"

"Clones?" Conrad screwed up his face.

"Unlikely," Anders responded. "Dolly the sheep took 277 tries."

"Not science fiction, for Christ's sake," Conrad rolled his eyes.

"If it is clones," Richard's deep voice framed the question. "Damn. Are you sure you have only two cases?"

"Six cases!" Conrad snapped. "Weren't you listening in my office?"

"We can't be certain unless we talk with Czajkowska," Anders said.

"Let me see," Conrad fumed. "Do I have this straight? Not only do we have an unknown number of children infected by a virus the CDC cannot cure, we also have a couple of dykes—both gene researchers—who cannot reproduce without male partners and instead used our clinic to implant cloned embryos into our patients?"

"Un-fucking-believable," said Richard.

"Exactly my point," said Conrad.

Anders didn't buy it. "If they had a lab, possibly. But to get an acceptable survival rate—I can't imagine it."

"I can," Richard said. "Suppose she did have a lab in the building," he looked into the distance as he spoke. Anders stared down at the faux-Elvis and let his imagination follow his words. "I can see her, wearing a white coat, working at a bench, studying a Petri dish." Richard looked up at Anders. "She has prepared embryos. She covers the Petri dish, stands, puts it in her lab coat pocket, and leaves."

"I don't like the sound of this," Conrad said.

"She smuggles them into the clinic during regular hours," Richard continued. "She enters the lab. Other technicians are there but, since she works there, they don't pay any attention. Theresa picks up a tray of Petri dishes, carries them to an incubator and places them inside."

"And?" Conrad prompted.

"She swaps her embryos for yours. With one hand, she slips a dish from the incubator into her lab coat pocket and replace it with the one she had hidden."

"Christ," said Conrad. "Who'd know?"

"No one," Richard said. "She closes the incubator door. The two technicians are engrossed in their own work and don't notice the swap."

Anders thought Richard's scenario was clever, but knew that making it work was vastly more complicated. "There are a lot of variables. You'd need the right number of embryos at the right stage of development. Keeping them alive? It would take meticulous planning. They would have to be highly skilled and highly motivated."

Conrad threw up his hands and stepped toward the restaurant.

"Sounds to me like a done deal."

Anders was closest to the door and held it open for them to enter. Richard strode into the restaurant and asked, as he passed, "What about Miss Czajkowska, the cloning expert in Amsterdam?"

Before Anders could respond, Conrad, who was following Richard, paused and surveyed him with a paternal air. "Anders, I want this problem to go away. So do you. Believe me, you do."

Anders suddenly recalled the feeling, as a junior officer, of being dispatched on a dangerous mission with ambiguous orders. Were their priorities viruses or clones? "What? I can't leave my patients."

"I don't see we have a choice," Conrad said. "We need two pieces of information: First, whether we're dealing with clones; second, and even more important, the genetic code so we can silence the RNA virus. No one else knows enough to question this woman. We'll watch the children. You go. And keep your goddamn pecker in your pants."

Anders didn't need to hear that and felt his back and shoulders stiffen. Conrad noticed his partner's discomfort. He stepped back, placed a hand on Anders' shoulder, and softened his expression.

"You'll be back in one day, Tiger."

~

The lower half of the Dutch door was wood, while the upper half was frosted glass. Anders read the black painted lettering at eye level: "Biotechnologische Studiereizen." *I hope she's back from lunch*, he said to himself. *No, you better hope she's reasonable.* Anders reached for the handle and pulled open the door.

He peered into a large space filled with natural light from a row of windows on the opposite wall and counted four lab benches covered with an assortment of beakers, pipettes, glass tubing, and workstations. Seated on a stool at the nearest table, a woman stared at him with palpable resentment. She wore a lab coat that didn't diminish the trendy appearance of her spiked hair, designer glasses, and leather boots, but did add a full measure of competence.

"Yes," she spoke Dutch. "Can I help you?"

Anders strode into the room with a raincoat in one hand and his other pulling a carryon. He responded in Dutch.

"My name is Doc—"

"Doctor van der Veer," the woman interrupted. "Yes, we met once in San Francisco."

Anders thought he would have remembered, but he couldn't place her.

"Sorry, I didn't recall." He moved toward her table. "Anne Czajkowska?"

She ignored the question.

"Why are you here? You must know about Theresa."

She wasn't giving him time to think. "Yes, I do. It was very sad. I'm here because I need your help."

"How could I possibly help you?" Her sarcasm was laced with contempt.

Very aggressive, he thought and realized he had to plunge into the freezing pond. Anders hung one butt-cheek over an empty stool next to her, draped his coat over his knee, and leaned in. Even sitting, he towered over her.

"We've got a situation at our clinic," he said.

Anne's expression didn't change. Her eyes looked up into his with an unrelenting gaze. She shook her head, slowly, inscrutably.

Anders couldn't believe she was this brazen. He returned her stare and waited. After a minute, her face grew tense. She stood, lips tight, and walked to another bench to remove the cover from a microscope.

"All right," Anders said to her back. "Our lab found matching DNA profiles in children whose embryos supposedly came from different parents."

Anne turned to face him with a thin smile. "Of course that is possible if they came from the same mother. What do you think?"

"My partner thinks they're clones."

Her mocking laugh dismayed him.

"Doctor, reproductive cloning is too risky. I don't have to tell you that." She dropped the instrument cover on the bench and walked around to the far side. Anders stood and caught up to her in three strides.

"The state of the art in reproductive cloning is well advanced," he retorted. "So far, no one has presented a live human for verification of cloning, but I wouldn't be surprised if you found a way to do it."

"If I did, if it was possible, so what?" her voice erupted with such venom that Anders stepped back. "The cloning genie is out of the bottle. We clone many mammals, including horses that are allowed to race so we can learn to improve the breed. But what of our human destiny? Cloning can be safe and effective. It should be considered a viable form of reproduction. Surely, a doctor in your field must agree."

Her fair skin was now bright red. Anders said nothing. He leaned against a lab table and waited for the anger to cool. It didn't take long.

"I don't agree that cloning is safe," he said. "We are looking at a 97 percent failure rate in bringing cloned embryos to term and many of those that do survive suffer health problems later."

"That rate is for scientists who are afraid to explore the process," she shot back. "They are afraid that cloning will threaten the human race by either diminishing the man's role in reproduction or introducing a population of super-humans."

Anders looked away, took a moment to get himself back on track, then faced her again. "I'm not here to debate the science or the ethics of cloning. Someday, it will be as commonplace as *in vitro* fertilization is now. But it is illegal in California, the home of my clinic, and I must know with certainty that clones were not implanted in any of my patients."

He watched Anne's face as her thoughts moved beyond the combustion point. She took a breath and flashed him a quick look of resignation. "I have experimented with cloning," she said. "It is true. But nothing like you imagine."

"You taught Theresa?" he asked.

"She could not manage. As you pointed out, the process is complicated and the failure rate is high."

Was that surprise or disappointment? Anders couldn't tell. Either way, he was relieved that she had almost eliminated a dangerous possibility.

"She didn't take it any further? What did she do next?" he wanted to be sure.

Anne stared at him with ice in her eyes. "She disappeared."

~

Anne was upset that Anders had entered her lab and provoked her anger. Why had she lost control? She wasn't jealous that he'd been with Theresa. He wasn't a nobody; he was a respected authority in his specialty. *So, why am I angry?* Then she realized it wasn't him. It was her. It was about her concealing her role in helping Theresa.

"These children," she heard him say. "Our lab found a gene sequence that belongs to a virus."

"I do not know about viruses."

"Could Theresa have engineered a disease? I mean—"

"No," she interrupted. Of course Theresa knew all about diseases and about gene manipulation, but that wasn't her interest. "She wanted to know about cloning."

"We have a ward full of very sick children."

"Theresa wanted to help me advance my theories."

"I think she used you," he said.

Anne saw his conviction. She thought back to the questions she had asked herself, the coincidences that had brought Theresa into her life. She knew. He knew.

Suddenly, she felt embarrassed. Her face flushed. Anger rose in her throat. "I cannot believe it."

"She used me also."

"Funny," she snapped at him. "Theresa said that about you. You stole her idea to increase the yield of fertilized ova."

"What?" His voice jumped an octave. His face turned red. "She only made a suggestion," he stammered. "I don't think she even knew the implication."

"Doctor, she was an expert in gene replication. She knew what she was saying and, on this topic, certainly more than you."

Anne saw that he would never accept that an assistant could know more than he did. *Proud man. We'll take him down.* She sat slowly on a lab stool.

"She also said you killed her unborn child—and yours. Did you really do that?"

The sudden flash of contempt is his eyes startled her.

"I'm a doctor. I help women have babies. I don't kill them."

"But she said—"

"She had an ectopic pregnancy." He was furious. "I did a Laparoscopy. Her fallopian tube was ruptured. There was no choice. She could have died. I explained all that, showed her the scans, but she insisted that I was only trying to save my marriage."

She was confused. She believed him. Until now she'd only heard Theresa's side of the story. But why had she lied? The answer rolled over her like a giant wave: so you would help her, of course. *Someone save me from myself.*

The alarm sounded from the mobile in her pocket. Her hand reached into her lab coat and switched it off.

"Sorry, Doctor. I must go now. I cannot miss this meeting with the director."

Anne stood and walked to the table where she had originally been sitting when Anders had entered her lab.

"Wait," he said. "You can't go until you tell me what she did."

She gathered her papers and bag, aware that the conversation was not finished and that Anders was watching her, expecting more. She felt sorry for him.

"I apologize. I have no time."

"Did she leave papers or notes when she left?"

If only he would shut up so I can go to my meeting, Anne thought.

"No," she said as she hurried toward the door. Then she realized she was being unnecessarily cruel. She stopped, grabbed a small notepad from her bag, and tossed it to Anders.

"Her mother may know something. Write your number. Leave it on the table. I will text you the address in Rome."

As she turned into the doorway, she saw Anders catch the pad and reach into his jacket for a pen. He gave her a skeptical look.

"What could her mother know?"

She was about to close the door, but held it open with one hand and leaned toward Anders.

"Why her daughter was such a manipulative bitch."

She let go and the door slammed shut.

~

The summer heat usually leaves Rome by October, but this year it lingered, waiting for the autumn breezes to carry it away.

Rotten luck, thought Anders. He had no summer clothes, intending only to visit Amsterdam, and was now hot and uncomfortable walking in wool slacks and a long-sleeve cotton shirt.

Thanks to Anne, he had found via dei Balestrari, a busy alley off Piazza Campo de Fiori and knew what Natalia Lanzatella looked like. He only needed to wait until Sunday Mass finished for Theresa's mother to pass through the alley on her way home.

Anders stopped in front of a trattoria. Inside, he saw a lone man in his fifties seated at a small table smoking and reading *Corriere dello Sport*. He wanted to watch people coming from the piazza and decided he could not do it from inside. The *tabaccia* adjacent had a display of newspapers and postcard on racks beside the entry. Anders regarded the papers for a long time. He spun a rack of postcards and periodically glanced over his shoulder to study the pedestrians. It was obvious to the crone seated behind the register in the doorway that Anders was wasting time. He caught her distrustful glare as he rolled up his sleeves in search of some relief from the soggy heat.

He started to move away, but spotted a woman sashaying up the narrow passage in a blue Sunday dress and matching handbag, giving cordial greetings to those seated or standing against the walls. It was her.

Anders moved toward the woman with his best smile and saw suspicion darken her face with every long stride he took. He addressed her in Italian.

"Scuzi, signora Lanzatella?"

When he reached her, he towered over the slight woman, though her step didn't falter and her Italian was curt. "Go away. I have no money."

"Madam, please," Anders pressed in Italian. "No money. I need to talk. I need your help."

"No money?" She slowed, but kept walking. Anders noticed her shrewd appraisal.

"What is your name, sir?"

"Doctor Anders van der Veer. Theresa used to work for me."

Recognition washed the suspicion from her face. "So. The

famous doctor of women. I have heard your name." She lengthened her stride, brushed past Anders, and flounced toward the trattoria.

"You may come. I take my coffee."

Anders followed her into the eatery and, while she stood proudly waiting at the bar, dropped some coins on the cashier's desk, took the receipts, and joined her. He let Natalia study him as he dropped the tiny papers on the white marble and nodded to the barrista.

"So, famous doctor, why are you here?"

"English?" he asked

Natalia rolled her eyes and then said, in English, "Even with your Dutch mouth, your Italian is excellent."

Anders smiled. The barrista set two espresso cups on the marble and slid the container of sugar in front of them.

"Very well," she said. "Tell me."

Anders had thought how he would approach Natalia, but still wasn't sure where to begin. He spooned two sugars into his coffee. Stirred it. "You know that the police believe Theresa drowned," he said.

Her dark eyes made him feel like a fool.

"Doctor, you did not come to tell me of my daughter. Speak."

All preparation in vain, he thought. *Very well.*

"Some of my patients are dangerously sick."

Now he saw she was perplexed. "But you. You are doctor."

"I don't know this disease," he said. "But Theresa did. If she kept records, they could save many lives. Did she leave any papers with you?"

"She leave nothing." Her haughty tone made the idea seem ludicrous.

Anders drank his coffee while he stared at her and tried to decide whether she was being truthful. In turn, she studied his skeptical expression, searching for meaning.

"She does not come here for long time."

He still doubted her. "I need whatever she left."

Natalia just smiled at him.

"I think you are not knowing my daughter, doctor." She drew the espresso cup to her lips, drained it, and turned to leave.

Anders followed her into the alley. She continued in the direction she had been going, but at a leisurely pace. Anders strolled beside her.

"For ten years, her father, that jackal, is living in Dubai." He could hear her bitterness. "Everyone there is criminal. All the time fight. One day he is driving and, boom." She claps her hands.

"Explosion?" he asked.

"Not so clever, eh? Theresa go to him. Stay long time. She meet big boss. He fall in love. Give her money. She study university."

This news surprised Anders, even more than the contempt in her voice.

"He see she is genius, this biotechnology. In France, they pay big money for her work."

Anders gazed at the flagstone and tried to digest what he heard. He thought he knew Theresa, but this was news. He felt Natalia watching him for a reaction. He kept his eyes on the stonework.

"You think you are too much man, Doctor."

Anders was slow to catch the new direction.

"Theresa say 'I love you,' no?" she asked.

He wasn't sure he wanted to go there and gave her a veiled stare. *She sees right through me.*

"Yes. I think so. But to boss man, she say, 'I die for you.'"

Anders understood her meaning and was about to answer when he saw a slight man leaning against a doorway push himself off the wall, spin, and hustle away. The motion caught Natalia's attention also and he saw her face sour.

"Oh no," she said and hurled a fist at the retreating figure. "Fottuto cane, lasciare del mio occhio." She spit emphatically on the flagstones.

"When The Jackal want to see what I do, he bring The

Weasel."

Anders understood and at the same time saw a change in Natalia.

"Okay." She said and turned to face him, apparently having reached a decision. "So. I tell you now. You want to know her work? You ask the father. Go Dubai. The Jackal has many eyes. He find you."

Natalia was facing him. He saw her place a forefinger below her right eye and pull down the lower lid.

"But look close, Doctor, you should go home alive, yes?"

~

Zaafir Ibrahim didn't mind that he had just dropped several thousand dollars in fuel, landing fees, and passenger services for a ten minute stop at the flight facility on Orly Airport. He had just collected the woman who he hoped would soon become his wife.

But he did mind the petrochemical stink of jet exhaust that burned his nose the moment he stepped out of the private terminal. His companion scrunched up her nose. She was equally miserable. Yet, in spite of the discomfort, he was content, feeling the joy of walking arm-in-arm with her across the tarmac beneath a clear evening sky in Paris. They could look forward to a smooth flight to Karachi.

Just thinking about his time with her on the plane filled him with anticipation. But as he stepped onto the narrow air-stair leading up into the gleaming jet, she withdrew her arm from his so she could follow behind. The movement distracted him. He felt his right shoe catch on the aluminum step. As he lurched forward, an image of impending pain flashed through his mind, then he felt strong hands grab his arm and pull him upright. He marveled at the strength of this small woman and silently rejoiced at his good luck in finding her.

~

The ruby grapes looked succulent. *The best fruit in Europe*, Anders thought. He gave the weathered woman beside the produce stand a five euro note and waited while she made change. He took the coins and tucked the grapes, which she had wrapped in newspaper, under his arm, stepped out from beneath the awning, and stood to admire the quaint fountain near the center of the Campo di Fiori.

In less than ten seconds the sun burned through his cotton shirt and propelled him into the dappled shade between the rickety stalls that vendors for the Sunday Market had setup to sell used house wares, illustrations torn from old books, broken furniture, scratched records, and other piles of unidentifiable junk.

Anders ambled between the booths under the grim scrutiny of vendors who hoped he was more than a tourist but knew better. The specific odor of rotting farm produce, garbage, and sewage brewed in the sun's growing heat reminded him of excursions he and Pryia had made to open markets in happier times. He sensed her presence beside him and waited for the sound of her voice. After a few more steps, his mobile chirped. Caller ID told him that Conrad had just saved him from another tongue lashing.

"Anders," he said into the phone.

"Anders," Conrad's voice was hollow. "I'm with Richard on speaker. How's Amsterdam?"

"Rome," Anders corrected. "You didn't get my message?"

"What the hell," Conrad said. "Fucking service! No. What's up?"

"Czajkowska gave me an address for Theresa's mother," Anders said.

Richard's baritone rumbled through the earpiece, "Is she a hot mama?"

Anders ignored the jibe and ambled away from the vendors' stalls toward a pillar of shade cast by the marble sculpture of sea nymphs rising from the pool in the circular fountain.

"They tried to use our patients for a cloning experiment," he said as he studied at the marble nymphs.

"Fucking lesbians. I knew it."

"It gets worse," Anders said.

"Christ."

"Theresa infected the children with viral RNA."

"The CDC was right," Conrad blurted.

"Yeah," Anders said. "And so were you. Way I figure it, with the new fertilization procedure? She could introduce it directly into the embryos."

"How?" asked Richard.

"I put her in charge of the lab."

"Jesus, Anders," Conrad fumed.

"What can I say? At the time, she was the best tech I'd ever met." Anders ripped open the newspaper around the grapes. "At least we don't have to worry about clones." He popped one in his mouth and asked, "How's Li coming with the frozen embryos? Has he found the gene sequence we need?"

"No," said Conrad. "Glick says we're out of time. Viral replication has started. The Davidson twins are still hanging on, but the others are getting critical."

Anders stopped chewing, felt a chill of anxiety run up his spine. "Start the critical patients on the Milwaukee Protocol. Emily knows what to do."

"Will do," said Conrad.

"While you're at it, ask the CDC why the mothers weren't infected. Blood from the fetus should have transported the virus and they should have displayed symptoms."

"Okay. I hadn't thought of that," Conrad said.

Anders focused on a table of tourists sweating under the sun in a *ristorante* across the piazza. "Shit, I hope she had files. We need to cure these children and prevent any contagion."

"Damn right!" Conrad said. "And those feeb nitwits want immediate quarantine. Keeler's nose is so far up my ass he can smell my toothpaste."

"They're saying it's—" Richard began.

Anders nearly choked, but managed to swallow in time to ask, "Bio-terrorism?"

"Torsloff thinks so," Richard said.

Conrad came on the line again. "Glick says two days. Then children start dying. That is unless your protocol works. What's your plan, sport?"

Anders didn't really have a plan. He was just following his nose. "Go to Dubai. See Theresa's father. Hope she left something with him."

"Rudy says she kept meticulous records," Richard boomed. "There must be a schema."

"But we gotta find it," Anders said.

"I know a guy in Dubai," Richard's deep voice was confident. "Name's Rahman. He can help. I'll have him contact you."

Anders wrapped the newspaper around the grapes and tucked the bundle under his arm. He turned away from the table of tourists and again faced the fountain. Leaning against the stonework that circled the pool of nymphs was the man Natalia had described as The Weasel. Anders glanced away and gave no sign of recognition.

"Good," he said. "I might need help. I'm being followed."

"Careful, partner," he heard Conrad's concern. "I don't want to see you on CNN wearing a blindfold."

Anders pocketed his mobile and ambled in the direction of the Weasel. As he passed the smaller man, Anders saw him avert his head. He took one more step, spun, and grabbed the Weasel's belt. Caught off guard, the Weasel did not resist as Anders forced him down onto the stone ledge and glowered into his eyes.

"Do you understand me?" Anders hissed in Italian.

The Weasel managed an impudent nod.

"Good," he said. "Tell Mister Parween I'll be in Dubai tomorrow morning."

The Weasel gave him a disdainful smirk.

~

Ibrahim pushed back into the white leather recliner in the cabin of his Gulfstream V and crossed his legs. He watched Faoud, his young bodyguard-steward, secure the boarding hatch and open the curtain that blocked the view into the cockpit during flight.

Despite his formidable size, Faoud moved in an aura of graceful intensity. He had already stowed Ibrahim's turban in the wardrobe along with his suit coat and Theresa's shawl. He brought them crystal glasses with ice and single-malt scotch.

As the aircraft began to roll, Ibrahim removed his tie and undid the top two buttons of his shirt. He took several deep breaths, reached for the crystal glass, and rolled a large swig of the smoky whiskey around his tongue. *Time to get a few things straight with my future wife,* he thought.

He regarded Theresa lounging in an identical seat, dark hair framing her face, dark eyes intent on the screen of the Macbook Pro on her thighs, lips pursed in concentration. He wanted to squeeze her, but that would come later. *How to begin?* he wondered.

"I am very happy to see you again. How was your time in Chennai?"

Theresa looked up from her computer. "Thank you, Uncle. I am happy to see you, too. I liked the meditation. It was calming. I did not like the spiritual teaching. I did not agree with it."

"You remained a long time," Ibrahim said. "I did not hear from you."

"I traveled. There was much to see. I needed to be alone." Her eyes returned to the computer screen.

He struggled to work up a scowl.

"I am not happy when you are away, child," he said in Hindi.

He saw her shrug. She continued to stare at the screen. Her fingers tapped the keyboard.

"I know, Uncle," she replied in Hindi. Then she added, with a touch of irritation, "It was necessary to advance my work with the virus. You agreed."

"I did," his tone was pleasant. "This once. But now, you stay. Leave business to me."

Theresa looked up and he felt himself melt in the warmth of her beautiful smile. "Did I not give you a clever plan to spread disease?"

He smiled back. "Very ingenious."

"Your clients did not pay well?" she asked.

He had to agree a second time. "Those fanatics paid dearly to feed their ambitions."

She gave another shrug, turned back to the laptop and adjusted the screen. "There, you see. You make me a scientist. I make you money. So, let me work."

She was going to drive him crazy. "Theresa, behave like a woman."

She looked at him again and beamed cheerfully, a taunting smile that seemed to say, "or what?"

Maybe this approach was too abrupt. Ibrahim changed the subject.

"Sanjay? Did he help?"

"Yes," she answered. "Thank you for him. He found the Dutch woman."

"You said she would be useful."

"Her technique was revolutionary," she explained. "But my idea to use clones was too difficult. So, I used frozen embryos from the doctor's clinic. Then, I let him believe he invented a new procedure." Ibrahim saw amazement spring forth in a sudden laugh. "He put me in charge of the lab. I could insert the virus directly into mother's embryo. No one would ever discover how it started."

Ibrahim nodded. He wasn't really interested in details. He gazed into his scotch and reflected on possible outcomes.

"Allah, may peace be upon him, will punish your personal vengeance."

Her hands withdrew from the keyboard, balled into fists and drove onto her hips. She gave him a bitter smile.

"Uncle, please. The man was false to me. I am right to destroy him. I used my knowledge to make a plan. When I saw it offered great potential for harm, I told you. Your clients paid for it. Everyone is happy."

"Still," he advised. "You must fight your enemies with a pure heart."

Theresa brought her hands together in front of her, intertwined her fingers and rested them in her lap. Her face grew somber and her eyes stared out the window.

After a few moments she said, "Sanjay made them believe I drowned. If the doctor should ever suspect—you can manage him. No?"

Ibrahim felt the warmth drain from his smile. He regarded her for a long time. Then he said, "You stay here, with me."

Skirmish

Anders could barely keep his eyes open. He didn't sleep on the flight from Rome and hadn't showered or changed clothes in three days. Sweat stung his eyes and the carryon he pulled along the jetway at Dubai International Airport hurt his shoulder. He followed the line of passengers out of a jet way into the brightly lit concourse. The PA system blared at him in Arabic.

He stepped out of line and stopped to gather his thoughts. From a crowd of greeters a man dressed in khakis approached him. His physique was imposing and reminded Anders of the Special Forces soldiers he'd treated in Afghanistan. The man's bass voice boomed at him in Dutch.

"Dokter van der Veer?"

"Ja."

"Welkom bij dubai."

"Good day to you, Mister—" Anders said in English.

"Ah so, English," the man said. He made no move to shake hands. "Gerrik van Vetter. I am to take you safely to Mister Parween."

Anders was too tired to be surprised. "That was fast."

"Not to worry, Doctor. I am in charge. He waved some papers in the direction of the main terminal. "This way. Immigration."

~

Anders heard the loud clang of the starting bell at Meydan Racetrack and saw a dozen Arabian horses burst from the starting gate on the far side of the track. The animals raced side by side down the back stretch, clumped together along the rail into the far turn and appeared in one thundering mass as they came out of the turn onto the straightaway to the finish.

Through the hot still air, Anders heard one race announcer speak Arabic; a second, English. In his seat by the handrail on the terrace of the Parade Ring Lounge, Anders leaned his elbows on the table overlooking the track and stared at the horses with zero interest. He was more impressed with the remarkable architecture of the world's largest and most expensive race track. The growing pitch of the crowd returned his attention to the race. The horses crossed the finish line and he heard van Vetter's voice beside him.

"Stront," came the curse. Anders watched van Vetter take the empty chair opposite. A waiter followed with a tray of Arabic coffee and shots of liquor. Van Vetter regarded the horses returning to the paddock and tore a race ticket into confetti. He dropped the pieces into an ashtray on the table. The waiter reached over his arm to serve their drinks.

"I prefer cockfights," he said to Anders.

Anders was bored. "Ever see Buzkashi?"

"Ah so, you were in Afghanistan," his tone offered a measure of respect. "Yes, a grim sport."

"More predictable." Anders gestured toward the track. Van Vetter reached one big hand for a shot glass while the other slid a second glass across the table to Anders.

"In the end, the goat is always dead."

"Waste of an afternoon," Anders agreed and took the offered glass.

"Enjoy yourself, please, while we wait for Mr. Parween to return. I will—" A movement in the paddock must have caught van Vetter's attention. Anders saw him stare in that direction with renewed interest. "Ah so. Someone I must see before the next race.

You remain here on the terrace, please. I will return in ten minutes."

Anders was falling asleep in the heat. He needed to move. "Think I'd rather walk around. I won't get lost."

Van Vetter gazed over the stands. He seemed to evaluate the chance of losing Anders in a place that seated sixty thousand. "There is much at stake here, Doctor. Do not wander far."

They both stood. "We meet here before the next race," van Vetter added.

Anders nodded. They both went into the lounge. Van Vetter turned in the direction of the paddock and Anders sought the exit leading down to the track. At the bottom of the stairs, the organic smell of freshly turned earth, much stronger than up on the terrace, refreshed Anders' senses. He pushed through the crowd—a mix of business suits, tourist shorts, and flowing white robes—most of them inspecting their favorite or potential favorite as the horses warmed up on the track. Anders soon noticed that someone in white kandura and keffiyeh had fallen in step beside him.

He turned his head and saw a tall man in his early forties with an attractive, swarthy face. The man smiled at Anders. He reached toward him with the back of one hand, but turned it over at the last minute to reveal a business card in his palm.

"Doctor van der Veer?" he said. "Abdul Rahman, inspector of customs services for the United Arab Emirates."

Anders took the card and read.

"Rahman." He was surprised. "How did you find me?"

"Your mobile," he said, still smiling.

Anders shook his head slowly. *Amazing*, he thought. "Technology. What you can do with it." He glanced at the card and put it in the pocket of his trousers.

When he faced Rahman again, he was unsmiling. The man took him by the arm and they walked with their backs to the Parade Ring Lounge.

"The one you are with, van Vetter. He should not see us together."

"He met me at the airport." Anders was puzzled. "He's taking me to see a Jana Parween."

This surprised Rahman. "You know Parween?"

"Not yet. His daughter worked for me."

Rahman glanced in the direction of the paddock as if to confirm they were not being observed.

"Mister Richard said you are seeking information to cure a disease at your clinic. It is very grave."

Anders nodded. "We think that Parween's daughter left information with him that could save many lives."

"I don't know his daughter, but you must be careful around this man."

"What do you mean?"

Rahman looked away and spoke in a low voice. "Jana Parween is small time," he said, looking at Anders. "But he works for a very powerful man. He was kicked out of India for bombing railways in Bombay—er, Mumbai."

Anders visualized a rail car exploding in a ball of flame. "Parween bombed a subway?" He was imagining Parween and his accomplice gloating over the explosion from a short distance away.

"No, no," Rahman corrected. "This man I'm telling you about is Ibrahim Zaafir. He is rich. His informants and cronies are everywhere."

"And Parween?" asked Anders.

"A smuggler. In the Gulf, it's a kind of gang war. Parween's car was bombed. You will see his face."

Anders stopped and leaned on a railing. He observed the jockeys and horses in matching silks. What was he getting himself into? Rahman leaned beside him.

"They are very secretive," the Arab said. "And very ruthless. If you should threaten their business, you will be food for the jackals."

Anders couldn't suppress a chuckle. "Funny. That's what Parween's wife calls him, The Jackal."

"Not funny, Doctor," Rahman cautioned. "If they decide to take you into the desert, you will not return."

They contemplated two horses walking back to the paddock. Rahman suddenly stepped back from the rail.

"Van Vetter is looking this way."

The man's vision amazed. Anders had seen nothing. Still he stepped away and let Rahman lead them into the crowd. After a few steps, Rahman turned back to him.

"If you suspect trouble while you are in Parween's home, you must call me."

"I'm not sure I'd recognize trouble," Anders said.

"Unusual activity, new faces, a change of venue." Rahman glanced again toward the paddock. "Van Vetter is returning."

He took Anders forearm in both hands and looked deep into his eyes with genuine concern.

"Call and I will help you, Doctor." Then he vanished into the crowd. Anders glanced toward the Terrace, but didn't see van Vetter.

However, as Anders reached the table on the terrace, he saw van Vetter standing beside it, craning his head, scanning the grandstands. When the Dutchman eventually spotted him, Anders saw that his eyes were full of suspicion.

"You got lost, Doctor," he accused.

Anders gestured at the crowd. "Must have just missed each other."

Anders sat and reached for a shot glass. Van Vetter stood for several moments watching him drink and then switched his gaze to the far side of the field so he could watch the horses enter the starting gate.

Anders heard a mobile ring and watched van Vetter withdraw it from the chest pocket of his safari shirt. His face showed no expression though Anders noted that he spoke in Hindi. Van Vetter finished and turned to him. His face was somber.

"I'm ready to take you to Mister Parween."

~

Anders felt alert for the first time in three days. Fresh from a shower, he lingered beside a credenza, sipped a glass of pilsner, and marveled at the unobstructed view of birds and fountains in the garden spread before him: Parween's estate. He smelled the cool perfumed air pass into the room behind him and decided that the garden view trumped both the impressive sculpture on the wall at his back and the golden Arabic script blazing from the marble walls to his right and left.

He had glanced briefly at the four armed guards motionless in the corners of the dining hall and the two servants waiting beside a Macassar ebony table that seated twenty-four, but was only set for two.

He stared at a framed photo on the credenza. It showed Theresa sailing through radiant blue water on some timeless ocean. He was fighting so hard to suppress the feelings it aroused that he almost didn't hear his host enter.

The scuffling of slippers and slow rhythmic clicking of a cane on the marble floor eventually penetrated Anders concentration. He raised his head and saw a very tall man limping toward him. He had dark skin and appeared to be in his mid-fifties, trim, and wearing a silk salwar chemise. But it was the man's disfigured face kept Anders spellbound longer than he knew was polite. He hoped it wasn't obvious.

"Doctor van der Veer," his voice had the timbre of a BBC radio announcer. "Welcome."

"Good evening, Mister Parween."

"Jana."

"Jana, yes." Anders gestured to the open wall. "You have a beautiful garden in the middle of the desert."

"Amazing, isn't it—what they do here with all their money." Parween gave a gracious smile. "You saw the race track."

Anders nodded and then gestured at the nearest guard. "You worry someone will steal the hors d'oeuvre?"

Parween's smile never faltered. "Security makes my guests feel at home. It relaxes them."

Anders nodded again, noncommittal, and turned to the credenza. "I was just admiring this photo of Theresa."

"One of my favorites," Parween drew close. "Taken while she studied in Marseilles."

Anders let Parween take his elbow in one hand and turn them toward the table.

"Doctor. Shall we eat?" He didn't wait for an answer. "Come. Let's sit."

One of the servants turned up at Parween's side and helped him to the head of the table. The other ushered Anders toward the seat on Parween's right. The glacial pace aroused Anders' anxiety.

"Jana, my time is very short."

Parween took his seat in silence. Anders followed and was immediately offered a hot towel by one of the servants while the other whispered in Parween's ear.

"Very well, Doctor," he said when the man finished. "But first, another beer or some wine with your dinner."

"Some wine. Thank you."

Parween nodded and the servant left the table just as others arrived with trays of food and drink. Anders could see the interview was going to take some time.

"Your wife doesn't think much of your activities," he said.

Parween sighed. "Ah well. Once, we were young and each of us was enchanted by the other's culture. I thought we could survive anything. But it was not to be. Natalia did not like the Middle East. Still, her family in Italy is well connected. So, after Theresa was born, I established her in Rome selling cigarettes."

That didn't sound like a favor to Anders. "Sorry?"

"By the boatload," Parween said, understanding the confusion. "Very lucrative. When Theresa was fourteen, well, my accident," he motioned to his face and leg. "Since this, Theresa came to live here and Natalia has never forgiven me."

Anders felt sympathy and tried to show it, but fatigue was returning while he sat. He gulped half of his wine when he meant to take a sip and banged the glass on the table when he meant to ease it down.

"She thinks you're a terrorist," he almost slurred.

Parween chuckled. "Seriously, she knows better. My activities make money, not converts."

"How so?"

"We broker goods and services. How people use them? Not our concern." It sounded trite to Anders.

"Some of my patients contracted a virus while Theresa worked at our clinic. I was hoping you might know something about her work?"

"I'm afraid not," Parween smiled. "The time has long past since I could understand what she did with her education."

"Did she ever study or work with viruses?"

Parween simply shook his head and appeared bemused. "Pity you came all this way, Doctor."

"I didn't set out to come here," Anders said. "We desperately need information. Theresa was the only one—"

Parween interrupted. "Doctor, perhaps you would consider the advice of an old Arabian fable."

Anders sipped his wine. He wanted to be tolerant.

"An old crane passes his days on the bank of the Euphrates, picking worms and insects from the mud," he began. Anders saw that Parween enjoyed the expressions and gestures of a natural storyteller and liked to regale his visitors.

"One day, he sees a diving hawk catch a lark in its talons. The crane is astounded. He decides to stop groping in the mud for worms. With his long legs and neck he will seek higher game. When a pigeon flies past, the crane launches himself in pursuit. He flies high, like the hawk, for a good dive. By the time he is high enough, the pigeon has landed on the river bank. Still, the crane dives. He breaks his long legs and neck on the ground."

Anders regarded Parween. "Not sure I follow."

"We say it is wise to be content with exercising your own special talents." Parween said it with a kind smile.

Anders considered the moral for several seconds, but a servant approaching the table distracted him. He watched the man walk up to Parween and then step to one side.

Suddenly Anders feared he was somewhere else. Insane. The wine, maybe. He was confused, couldn't trust his eyes. He saw a woman in Muslim dress, a shawl and head scarf. She had walked unseen behind the servant. He flashed on Theresa but it couldn't be her. *She's dead*, he thought. Anders felt his jaw drop and his legs fight to lift him from the chair. He wanted to jump up and shout, "Is it really you?"

"Theresa?" he blurted.

She gave him a vulnerable look. "Hello stranger."

She stopped beside Parween. Anders gaped at them. She removed the scarf, held it in one hand, and placed the other on Parween's shoulder. She looked down at her father.

"Hello, Papa. Sorry I do not call. Time was short."

Parween raised his head to look at his daughter. Anders could see embarrassment even though his dark complexion.

"I thought you were in Karachi."

"I was, Papa. Uncle sent me home. Thanks God. I am away from his whining women."

Anders could not speak. He regarded them, awestruck. Parween and Theresa exchanged a knowing look.

"I've just been entertaining your friend here. He's been searching for you. Thinks you have something he wants."

Theresa gave Anders a flirtatious look. "Anders? Oh, he always know where to find me."

"Apparently he does," said Parween and then noticed that Anders was still on his feet. "Oh Anders, please, have a seat." He turned back to Theresa. "Did Gerrik drive you?"

Anders slumped, dazed, into his chair.

"Yes, but he leave again," Theresa said. "You would know where he goes."

Parween switched to Hindi. "Yes, to the boat in Muscat. What did Uncle say?"

Theresa's eyes were on Anders, but her voice replied to Parween in Hindi: "My scent should fill his nose while Uncle finishes business with the Iranians and then decides what to do with him."

She smiled at Anders.

"How did he find you here?" Parween asked.

"It is a mystery and I am shamed by his presence." The smile hid the rancor in her voice. "But you know Uncle. We must play our role."

Theresa switched back to English. "Sorry, Anders. We finish some family business."

"S'okay." He was struggling. *What's going on?* His mind was racing. *Why isn't she dead?*

Parween picked up the conversation with his daughter in English. "Shall I ask Jamaal to fix you something?"

"I eat before. Thank you."

Theresa walked casually around Parween and took the chair beside Anders. "I just sit here with my friend, Anders."

She gave him another flirtatious look. "You are still my friend? No?"

Anders turned to her with a confused expression and said nothing.

Parween placed his palms on the table and pushed his chair back. Two servants rushed to help him stand.

"Well, in that case."

"Papa!" Anders heard the alarm in her voice.

"It's all right," he replied. "I have some business before I retire. You two go on."

Anders and Theresa rose as Parween shuffled away with help from the servants.

"Good night, Papa," she called after.

"Good night," said Anders and then he felt Theresa slip her arm through his and gently lead him toward the open wall to the garden beyond.

Underneath the night sky, a breeze occasionally fluffed her dark hair. Anders wasn't sure whether he was smelling flowers or Theresa's perfume. He felt heat where she held his arm and didn't know what to do next.

"Anders, my surprise to see you here. Did you not bring your wife?"

She liked to taunt. He ignored it. "I can't believe you're alive. Everyone thinks you drowned."

Her voice was coy. "Why do they think that?"

"You disappeared. The police found a body. But you're—how did this happen?"

She snuggled closer to Anders. "Does not matter, now. You see. I am here."

Anders felt joy, relief. He glanced at the urban sky, but saw no stars. "I would never have dreamed..."

His eyes descended to the orange skyline. "But, you've got to help. We have sick patients. They will die in two days."

He finally stared down at Theresa and the elation drained from him as if someone had pulled a plug. He stopped, drew his arm away, and faced her head on.

"Diseased children. In different cities. All from our clinic. We ran DNA tests. Some of them have the same mother."

She smiled, unconcerned. "How can that be?"

"You tell me." He waited while she thought for a moment, regarding him without guile.

"Perhaps many children are sick, but you hear only about children from your clinic. Maybe DNA tests are no good. You always tell me about contamination."

"Stop." Anders' disappointment rose in his throat. "Anne told me about your experiments, the cloning."

She guffawed, but he didn't pause.

"She said you wanted to switch your clones for the embryos I give my patients."

Her laugh was cheerful. "Don't talk crazy, Anders."

He pressed ahead. "Theresa, what did you do to my children?"

She leaned very close. He wanted to pull away. She reached up and put her hands on his shoulders and her eyes burned into his.

"Your children? I care for them. I protect them since they are alive only a few seconds." Anders felt her hands tremble, heard the intensity swell in her voice. "I work in your new lab to make them healthy. I help them back into their mothers. What you want me to say?"

She withdrew her hands and dismissed him with a sharp wave. She did a swift pirouette, walked a few steps and stood facing away with her hands on her hips.

"No more. Okay?"

Her anger cleared his head. He came here for a reason. With a purpose, a timeline. He stepped closer so he could face her again.

"What were you thinking?"

Her eyes flashed. "Technology, Anders. Can make woman equal to man." Her face filled with insolence.

"Infecting unborn babies? Killing innocent children?"

"It was not like that."

"I need to cure this virus, Theresa."

"Like you cure my pregnancy? Thanks to you, I can never have child."

He didn't believe she was serious. "Theresa, you know better."

She turned and walked slowly to a fountain. After a few moments, she lowered the shawl from her shoulders and leaned back on the stone. Her eyes found his and he saw she was relaxed, her eyes radiant. Her voice softened.

"You do something for me?"

Anders knew this dance. He moved closer, and kept his eyes dull.

"I need you to tell me about this virus," he repeated.

With one hand, Theresa teased the hem of her dress. Her left eyebrow arched and her lips drew a lopsided grin.

"Are you the same old Anders?" Her flashing eyes reached into his soul, hoping to incite his once ravenous desire, but this evening they could no longer tempt him. He knew what he needed. He stepped forward and took her shoulders in his hands.

He held her eyes for a long time. "Theresa, tonight. Tonight, I need answers."

She snapped back as if he'd poured water on her head. Her flat eyes continued to look into him, searching. Then, she reached one hand up to his face, her fingers touched his temple.

"So. You do bring your wife."

~

A servant had escorted Anders to the guest bedroom. It was dark and cool, the bed huge. He could have slept until Tuesday, but a steady knock tugged at the fabric of his dreamless world until it fell away and he lay naked wondering where he was. He opened his eyes, turned his head, and saw Pryia laying next to him propped up on one elbow, her abundant curves tempting beneath a white silk nightgown. He flinched.

She smiled. "Anything you want to say?"

He struggled to gather his thoughts and her image faded, replaced by red numerals on a clock: "12:30." *My God, I've only slept for an hour.*

The knocking, tapping, whatever, beat again in his ears. He sat up, threw a shirt on, and opened the door. Theresa gazed at him from the hallway. She wore safari clothes and her hair in a pony tail. Her voice was friendly but her eyes were sober.

"Sorry to disturb you."

Anders shrugged, still not awake, and waited for the explanation.

"Uncle is flying to Paris today. He will drop us in Rome."

His first thought was relief at the prospect of leaving, but then he asked, "Why?"

"I will visit mother and you will return to San Francisco."

He felt his thoughts come together. "Theresa, I still need information from you."

"There is time on the plane," her eyes softened, but her tone was more insistent. "We meet Uncle in Muscat. Is a five hour drive. We must leave now."

"All right. Give me a minute."

Theresa nodded. Anders retreated into the room and closed the door.

Now he was fully awake. He threw his few garments into the carryon, and then sat on the edge of the bed and took Rahman's business card from his pocket. He dialed his mobile and waited. The inspector answered on the second ring.

"This is Doctor van der Veer," he said into the phone. "They are taking me into the desert."

Assault

There is nothing like the quiet of a desert night, thought Ibrahim, now that Otto had shut down the G-5's engines. He waited calmly beside the aircraft with his trusted bodyguards, Faoud and David. The two men paced attentively on the landing pad that was located north of Muscat International's only runway. Ibrahim faced south toward the main terminal. All appeared well. He saw no activity in the predawn and, in any case, knew that the men in the tower were paid well to ignore his presence.

He wasn't sure what made him turn and face north toward the Gulf of Oman. He searched the glow above the hills, the mantle from the mercury vapor lamps along the coast highway beyond, but saw nothing.

Then his ears caught the thumping of a helicopter. He thought it must be coming from the Gulf, skimming over the desert. The thumping changed frequency and seemed to rise above the glare of airport terminal.

When he finally spotted it. Ibrahim saw the chopper execute a sweeping 90 degree right turn and descend straight for the him. He spun around and searched the frontage road paralleling the runway, saw two sets of headlights speeding toward him from the East. It's going to be a race.

Ibrahim shouted for Otto to start the engines, for the two porters carrying luggage from a car nearby to hurry and for Faoud and David to be ready for an assault.

In the cone of light from the aircraft's open hatch, Ibrahim and his bodyguards regarded the two Mercedes limos racing over the dirt road in front of them, listened to the helicopter descending behind them, and silently implored the cars to go faster.

In the back seat of the second limo, Anders sat beside Theresa. They were tearing across the desert and Anders' stomach rebelled at the dizzying speed, the rough road, and the lack of sleep. In addition, Rahman's warning had spiked his anxiety. He fought the nausea by staring past the driver and Parween and out the windshield.

Ahead of them, he glimpsed van Vetter in the lead limo stick his head out of the passenger window and look up at the sky ahead. Then he drew back inside and said something to his driver.

"What's he doing?" Anders asked.

"See that helo," Parween said pointing to the sky. "He's telling the driver to get there before that helo does."

"Why is he worried?"

"It's nobody we know," Parween said and lowered his head so he could follow the helicopter's path through the window. "Nobody we want to know."

Anders had no clue where they were. He was wondering how much farther when out his left side window, he saw a forty-foot ocean container beside the road.

Suddenly brake lights from the lead limo turned the haze in front of them red. Anders felt the brakes slam and the limo skid through the gravel. He braced for an impact, but the driver feathered the pedal and stopped them well shy of collision.

After a moment the dust cleared enough to reveal an armed man in camouflage fatigues standing in the road ahead of the lead limo with his right hand raised in a command to halt. His left hand wrapped around an automatic weapon—Anders instinctively recognized the Kalashnikov—that hung from his shoulder.

"What is this?" Parween said.

"Someone you know?" Theresa asked.

"No," said Parween.

Through the still swirling dust, Anders saw van Vetter open his door and step out. He held an MP5 machine pistol low behind the door where the armed man could not see it.

"Whatever it is, Gerrik will take care of it," Parween said.

Anders gut tensed. He didn't take his eyes off van Vetter.

"Who could it be?"

"Out here? Anybody," said Theresa.

Anders watched the armed man shout at van Vetter in Arabic. Van Vetter shouted back in Arabic. The armed man shouted again with greater authority and took a determined step toward van Vetter.

The Dutchman remained behind the opened door but shouted again and waved at the man to leave the road.

The armed man continued to advance and shout at van Vetter.

"Uh-oh." Theresa said.

"Patience, daughter. Gerrik knows what to do," Parween's voice was calm.

"He looks—" Anders started to say, but a movement out the window to his left distracted him. He saw four more armed men move into view from behind the ocean container.

Van Vetter must have seen them at the same time, because he raised his weapon and fired a short burst at the man in the road ahead.

The man lurched backward from the impact and fell in the road. A chorus of shouts arose instantly from the left and a volley of lead strafed both vehicles. Van Vetter stepped quickly onto the running board of limo and returned fire over the roof.

The rear doors of the lead limo flew open. Two soldiers scrambled out, firing at the assailants. At the same time, Anders saw his own driver throw open the door, jump out with an AK-47, then dance herky-jerky, and fall to the ground dead before he fired a single round.

That's when his world downshifted to slow motion. As he

turned to his companions, he imagined he saw a streak of smoke come from the desert on the right. The lead limo exploded in a glorious red-orange ball. The bodies of van Vetter, his driver, and the two soldiers spun in the roiling smoke like shredded dolls.

"Papa!" shouted Theresa.

Anders grabbed the AK-47 by Parween's seat and swung his body left to fire through the side window at the men by the road. He pulled the trigger and felt the concussion in the confined space slam his entire body. Glass flew everywhere. One man fell in the road and suddenly the limo surged. Anders snapped his head around and saw that Theresa had lunged forward into the empty driver's seat. She jammed the gear shift, spun the steering wheel left, and stomped the accelerator. The driver's door slammed shut and Anders almost fell backwards. They swerved and barely missed the smoking hulk of the lead limo. She plowed into two assailants and then accelerated through the bullet-laden dust toward the aircraft a hundred feet ahead.

The limo fishtailed violently as it gained speed, which kept more bullets from striking them, but also hindered Theresa's ability to steer for the G-5. Through the windshield, Anders saw two bodyguards kneeling beside the air stairs, shooting at the armed men behind. Suddenly, Theresa's head snapped forward onto the steering wheel.

The limo skidded to stop a few feet from the aircraft.

"Theresa!" Parween screamed.

Anders reached for Theresa. He barely heard bullets ping into the car or felt shattered glass spray the back of his head. He wanted desperately to help Theresa and didn't see a man sprint from the aircraft to the car and yank open the driver's door. But he did see him pull Theresa's limp body into his arms. He shouted for him to stop. The man ignored him, lifted the unconscious woman from the limo, spun around, and ran for the aircraft.

Anders turned to Parween, but he had already pulled himself out the passenger door and was hopping around the front of the car after the man with his daughter.

"Theresa!" he cried.

Anders felt himself yanked out the rear door and slammed to the ground. A face loomed over him and screamed above the din of automatic weapons fire. "Run to the plane!"

Adrenaline. Now he was all present. Cool gravel under him. A large sweaty man over him. Engine noise, gunfire, bullets whistling close. He scrambled to his feet, weapon in hand and sprinted for the air stairs, hurdling a man lying prone in his path, shooting at their assailants.

To his right, several men ran toward him from under the spinning rotor of a helicopter. He fired. One fell, one stopped. Two other men saw him, dropped the luggage in their hands, and fled.

He saw Parween ahead, part way up the air stair, moving fast for him, but not fast enough for Anders. As his right foot landed on the bottom stair, he felt a heavy thump in the back of his right thigh. The leg started to collapse, but he grimaced and pushed off with a loud groan.

Parween turned at the sound. Anders saw him go limp and pitch forward down the steps on top of him. The additional weight forced him to his knees. He dropped the weapon and with both hands struggled to control Parween's body. Finally, with a tremendous grunt, he straightened his legs and pushed them up the stairs into the cabin.

He found a place to lay Parween on the carpet. Behind him, the man who had taken Theresa ran to the open hatch and shouted, "David! Faoud! Let's go!"

Faoud bounded past the man into the cabin. "David is dead," he announced. "We can leave. Men from the helicopter are close."

The man stood just inside the hatch with one hand poised by the lever to retract the air stair and close the hatch.

"Otto, go, go, go," he shouted and grabbed the lever. Before he could pull it, one edge of the hatch exploded, hit by a spray of bullets, and drove fragments of lead and aluminum into the man's face, neck, and chest. Anders watched him fall backwards into the aircraft.

Faoud didn't hesitate, "Otto, now! Now!" He yelled and pulled the lever closing the hatch. The engines spooled up and they started to roll.

~

It's curious how trivia distracts you under stress. The hand-woven silk carpet in the Gulfstream's forward cabin was finer than any Anders had ever seen. He couldn't begin to guess at its value, with or without the blood stains.

Faoud knelt over the unconscious man who'd been wounded in the hatchway. Tears streamed down the big man's face. His hands moved helplessly in circles above the body, not knowing how or whether to touch him.

Parween lay in pain, unattended. He groaned periodically, loud enough to overwhelm the sound of the engines.

Anders was still pumped. He bent over Theresa and examined her bloody head wound. The pain in his leg hindered his movement, frustrated his thought process.

"I need medical equipment," he shouted, then looked at Faoud. "I can save her but I need medical equipment."

Faoud stared at him with pleading eyes, "You are doctor?"

"Yes, I'm a doctor."

Faoud pointed toward a stand of mahogany lockers that covered the port side of the cabin. "We have supplies. There."

Anders grimaced and pushed to his feet. He limped to the cabinet, yanked open one drawer, rummaged through it, another drawer, rummaged through it. He found most of the supplies he needed. "Where are the antibiotics? The medication?" he shouted, his voice full of tension.

Faoud raised his head and pointed. "Drawer. Down."

Sure enough. He piled everything into his arms and limped back across the cabin to Theresa.

"Wait," said Faoud when he saw where Anders was headed. "That is for Mister Ibrahim."

Anders kept moving, kept his eyes on Theresa. "In a minute. This is more urgent."

"No. Stop," the bodyguard commanded. He wasn't used to

being disobeyed. "It is for Mister Ibrahim. You must save him first."

This time, Anders glared at the imposing, if naive, Faoud. "His wounds can wait. This girl will die if I don't stop the bleeding right now."

Anders knelt beside Theresa. He couldn't see the threat in Faoud's eyes. "You will care for Mister Ibrahim. Leave her alone."

"She will die," he said and placed the surgical items on the carpet. He saw Faoud's hand flash like a snake and felt his throat in a strangling grip. He was pulled over Theresa's body until his face was inches from the bodyguard's.

"You will die," Faoud spat. He thrust Anders toward Ibrahim. "If Mister Ibrahim die, you die."

With the vise on his throat, Anders could barely squeak. "She will die before Ibrahim."

Faoud released Anders, drew his automatic pistol, and held it to Theresa's head.

"Yes. She will die now," Faoud was emphatic. Anders didn't believe it until he looked into the man's eyes.

"Stop. Wait. All right. Is there a bed? Someplace I can work?"

"Work here. Start now," he was relentless.

Anders picked up a scalpel and cut into Ibrahim's shirt so he could examines the chest wounds. He saw a couple of nasty tears on the left side over his ribs and hoped the fragments had not penetrated his lungs. There were serious but not life-threatening injuries to his face and neck. He tore open a syringe, reached for a bottle of anesthesia, and inserted the needle.

Faoud watched him. "What is that?"

"Anesthetic."

"No," the bodyguard said. "No anesthetic."

"This will be painful."

"No anesthetic," he insisted.

Anders eyed Faoud, but spoke gently as he would to a child. "You want me to save him? I must be very careful. He cannot move while I work."

"He will be asleep?"

"Yes."

"Okay. Anesthetic," Faoud relented.

Anders found a vein in Ibrahim's arm and injected the fluid. He unwrapped a scalpel and clamps, tore open packets of gauze, and began to repair the wounds.

~

Rahman stepped from the helicopter onto the warm tarmac of the North Landing Pad. The rotors had stopped. He caught the suffocating smell of jet exhaust and cordite mixed with burning rubber from the smoldering limo. The previous day's heat still hung in the early hour.

Fifty feet away a police major and two of his officers stood over a prone body on the landing pad where the G-5 had been. They were watching the jet ascending into the deep purple dawn. They were probably thinking the same thoughts that troubled him: the helicopter pilot had landed too far from the jet for his men to reach it in time.

The major seemed transfixed, watching the plane's blinking lights vanish into the night. One of the officers stepped to the corpse and rolled it face up with his foot. The other joined him and spit on the body. Rahman watched both men spit and kick it with growing contempt.

"Wait," he shouted and hurried toward them. "Stop. Let me see who it is."

The policemen backed away as he approached. Rahman studied the corpse then shook his head in dismay. He moved a few steps until he stood beside the major. They contemplated the receding aircraft in silence.

~

Parween could find no relief from the burning in his body. At least the car bomb had rendered him unconscious. Drugs had soothed him in the hospital afterward. But this? Lying on the carpet of the G-5, there was no escape. The rhythm of agony, an intense wave of mind-shattering pain that forced him cry out, tormented him longer than he could bear. Then, the mystery. The gut wrenching would subside from intolerable, but no matter how hard he wished it to stay away or tried to control his body, the torture always returned as strong as ever.

He was breathing hard, he knew it. He tried to slow down, opened his eyes. He saw Anders kneel beside him. The man didn't seem well, but still he lifted Parween's salwar chemise and examined his wounds.

Parween could barely speak. "Doctor, my daughter?"

"Head wound." His impassive expression told Parween the news was bad. "Hard to say."

"Will she?"

"Possibly, yes."

Parween whispered again, "Ibrahim?"

"He'll be all right."

He felt the doctor adjust his salwar chemise and put something beneath his head as he spoke. "I'm a little concerned about you, though."

Parween wasn't worried about himself. "Ibrahim will never forgive if Theresa dies."

"You just take it easy, Jana," he said in a comforting voice.

Parween struggled to make him understand what was at stake. "I gave her life. He gave her—" He saw the doctor nod and wait for him to continue. But the words would not come. The thoughts would not come. He saw only one thing as his vision faded. "I...mother—"

~

Rahman lit the major's cigarette and then his own. The policeman admired his Zippo briefly before turning to watch his staff tend the wounded on the North Landing Pad.

"What about the weapons?" he asked, keeping his eyes on the policemen.

"Gone. Across the strait two days ago."

"And the cash?"

A line of policemen filed past them carrying dead and wounded comrades to vehicles waiting on the concrete. The sight angered Rahman.

"Still on the plane with that piece of camel shit. No thanks to your men."

When the major turned to him, he could see the man was offended. "You told us to hurry. I said we didn't have enough men. What did you want me to do?"

"Stop the plane," Rahman barked.

"We did our best. Look what it cost us."

Rahman shut his eyes. He knew it wasn't the major's fault. The pilot had landed in the wrong spot. The attempt to stop the limos had been weak because they didn't have enough men and weapons. He'd been forced to initiate the operation at the last minute. The whole thing happened too fast. He faced the major.

"I am sorry for your men," Rahman said. "For all our sakes, I hope we catch the plane in Rome."

~

Anders sat on the small bench in the Gulfstream's aft cabin and regarded Theresa and Ibrahim's unconscious bodies on the double bed. The man would be okay; the woman, he wasn't sure. He had tended them carefully, sutured Ibrahim's face, neck, and chest, ensured that his lung was undamaged; cleaned and bandaged Theresa's bleeding head wound. After that, he had taken time to dress his own wounded leg. No vascular or skeletal trauma. He'd survive. Poor Parween, though. He'd begun to like the old thief.

When Ibrahim stirred, Anders rose and limped to the bed. He sat beside his patient and waited until his eyes fluttered open.

"Sir," he inquired. "How is your breathing?"

"Uh."

Still groggy from the anesthetic, Anders concluded. "You're going to be okay. Just take it easy."

Ibrahim opened his mouth and winced. He closed it and rolled his eyes. He tried his mouth again, gingerly and asked in a hoarse whisper, "Theresa?"

"She is alive."

Ibrahim fumbled around behind him with one arm. When he finally felt Theresa on the bed, he attempted to roll over and face her. Anders placed on hand gently on Ibrahim's shoulder to restrain him. He didn't want the man to irritate his wounds.

Ibrahim objected. "I need her."

"Yes," Anders acknowledged.

Ibrahim looked at him. "She is the spice in my life." Tears came to his eyes. He grew agitated. "She is stubborn. Look at her now. A woman should be at home."

Anders nodded hoping to calm him.

"Faoud?" Ibrahim asked

"Asleep. Do you want him?"

Ibrahim's nod was barely perceptible.

Anders pressed up off the bed and limped to the forward cabin. Parween's corpse lay covered on the carpet. Faoud slept in one of the lounge seats. Anders limped to him and tapped his shoulder. His eyes snapped open. He nodded to Anders and rose from his seat.

In the aft cabin, Faoud knelt beside the bed while Anders observed from behind. He didn't understand Hindi, but their body language and use of proper names led him to conclude that Ibrahim had asked whether Theresa was alive. Faoud had said she was, but Parween was dead. He wasn't sure about the rest of the exchange, but it sounded like Ibrahim had asked about Anders' role and Faoud had responded that he had saved their lives.

Ibrahim seemed to contemplate Anders while he caught his breath. Then he appeared to give Faoud instructions for Otto because Faoud rose and headed to the cockpit.

Ibrahim glanced at Anders and patted the bed beside him. "Sit here."

"Are you having much pain?" Anders asked as he lowered himself to the mattress.

"I'm fine. But I see fuzzy."

"It's the anesthetic."

Ibrahim had recovered his senses. "You have done great service. Saved Theresa and me. Our lives."

"I am a doctor." To Anders it was self-evident.

Ibrahim had a gracious expression. "At least I can repay you in kind. I instructed Otto to take us to Paris."

"What about Rome?" Anders was puzzled. Was this better or worse for him?

"Nasty surprises in Rome." Ibrahim scoffed. "For you, Paris is healthier."

"But—" he couldn't think fast enough.

"You will still have your ticket to San Francisco," Ibrahim assured.

"I don't have what I came for," Anders said.

"What is that?" Ibrahim was deliberate.

"Theresa. Information to save my patients."

"Theresa cannot go with you." He regarded Anders for several moments. "However, I was told of certain things in your clinic."

At last, thought Anders. *Answers.*

"Now, you save my life. I am truly sorry for the trouble they will cause."

"Trouble already," Anders admitted.

Ibrahim had recovered quickly from the anesthetic, but was now running out of strength. His head started to nod. "Unfortunate. It is done. I am honor-bound not to interfere."

"But my patients." Disappointment overcame Anders. His tone grew pleading. "Theresa has information that will save them."

"For your patients, I am also sorry. As for Theresa—" His hand moved slightly to indicate her lying beside him. "You can see for yourself."

"Sir, you can't—"

Ibrahim raised a finger and Anders immediately felt Ibrahim's power.

"Doctor, I can. I must." He closed his eyes.

Anders knew Ibrahim was out for the count. For a long time, he studied the sleeping man and the unconscious woman who had created havoc in his clinic, his life. Frustration spread through him. *I've come so far*, he thought. *Yet I don't know any more about solving this crisis than when I started.*

Anders moved to the foot of the bed and sat with his elbows on his knees and his head in his hands. *How can I possibly find Theresa's notes?* He wondered. *I'm running out of options.*

He felt his body shaking. He dropped his hands and his torso swayed forward and back. He rolling his head in circles trying to loosen the knots in his neck and shoulders. As his head rolled right, his eyes fell upon a soft leather bag by the foot of the bed. It lay open, with a corner of brushed aluminum protruding through the zipper.

He froze. He couldn't move for several seconds. Then he was shaking with excitement. He shot a look into the forward cabin and saw Faoud's feet in the nearest recliner.

Anders leaned over and grabbed the MacBook Pro. He held it to his chest. It wouldn't fit under the shirt and it was too big to be concealed in his pants. *I need another way*, he thought.

He turned the computer over and examined the latch for the battery cover. A noise came from the forward cabin. Was Faoud awake? He looked at the door, but could no longer see his feet.

Anders knelt on the cabin floor. His hands, steady during the most harried surgery, now shook almost beyond control. He willed his fingers to remove the cover and lift out the battery. Underneath, a retaining bar securely held the hard drive. He heard clanking in the forward cabin.

My only chance, he told himself. Stay calm. Reaching into a pile of trash he grabbed a scalpel and unscrewed the plastic retaining bar. His fingers lifted the drive and placed it on the floor. He didn't bother with the retainer, but dropped the battery into place, snapped on the cover and slid the laptop into the bag just as Faoud appeared in the door and saw him on the floor.

"What are you doing?"

Anders dropped a bloody towel over the hard drive and held the scalpel toward Faoud. "Just cleaning up."

Faoud's eyes searched his for several seconds before leaving the doorway. Anders snatched the bloodstained drive and shoved it into his pants pocket. He tried to breathe. He couldn't stop shaking.

~

Anders had flown often to Charles de Gaulle and found Terminal 2E with no trouble. Now past customs and immigration, he limped by the carnival of duty free shops. The only crowd in a boarding area led him to the San Francisco departure. He checked his watch; time was short. The mobile in his jacket chirped. *Perfect*, he thought and snatched it from his pocket.

"Anders," he said, wondering who would be calling from the Emirates.

"Good morning, Doctor." Of course.

"Rahman!"

"Where are you?"

"Paris, at the airport."

"We lost you," Rahman said. Anders thought he sounded disappointed, but didn't have time to analyze it. He had joined the last few passengers lined up for the flight and noticed several men staring at him. He lowered his head, spoke in a hushed voice.

"There was an ambush at the airport in Muscat and we flew to Paris."

"Not an ambush, Doctor. The police."

"Everyone thought they were thieves," Anders said.

"The police went to save you and to arrest Parween and van Vetter."

"It was very grave," Fresh memories brought back the sadness.

"Yes," Rahman sounded empathetic. "Van Vetter is dead. What about Parween?"

"One second," Anders stopped for the gate agent holding out his hand. He tucked the phone onto his shoulder and surrendered his boarding pass, watched the agent scan it. No smile. Anders headed for the jet-way.

"Also dead," he resumed. "Theresa has a head wound."

"Were you hurt?"

"I'm okay."

Now in the jet-way Anders saw he was the last passenger hurrying to the aircraft.

"I'm glad you are safe. Will the girl survive?" Rahman asked.

"She may—but a different life."

"We wanted the airplane."

"No one knew what was happening," Anders said.

"Parween delivered a boatload of weapons to Kereti across the Gulf of Oman two days ago," Rahman explained.

"What, in Iran?" Anders sounded surprised.

"Yes," Rahman continued. "We heard his boss collected three billion dollars. They were flying it to France. I thought Ibrahim might be aboard. Did you see him?"

"I saved his life. He was wounded in Muscat." Anders had taken several steps before Rahman answered.

"I suppose you had no choice."

The line of passengers was moving quickly. Anders neared the aircraft hatch. "Sorry, Rahman. I'm just about to board—" The signal cutoff.

Anders didn't bother to remove the phone from his ear as he presented his boarding pass. This entitled the purser to scowl at him, glance at the stub, then gesture for Anders to stow the device, and hurry up (please) to his seat.

~

Anders didn't know which feeling caught up to him first, fatigue or sorrow. He stared out the window of seat 54-J, on Air France flight 410, drew the blanket tighter under his chin, and tried to push the last twenty-four hours from his mind.

He could not chase away his feelings. Someone watching would have seen waves of conflicting emotion cross his face. He held the hard drive in one hand. He turned it over and studied the bloody fingerprints. His eyes welled with tears. He dried them with the blanket, but they kept coming. He dabbed at his eyes again. It did no good. Eventually he gave up, laid his head back and let it all flow.

He wanted to talk to Pryia.

~

An eight-hour nap on the flight snapped Anders out of his funk. He strode into his partner's office. Conrad and Richard stopped talking when they saw him.

"Anders!" Conrad offered a brusque greeting. "I said one day, not three."

Richard was only somewhat kinder. "Mr. Intrepid," he said with a smile.

Anders said nothing. He walked to them, removed the hard drive from his pocket, held it up in one hand and waggled it back and forth with his wrist.

"The goods, gentlemen."

Richard was nonplussed. "You found Theresa's laptop?"

Anders bowed fifteen degrees. Richard smiled and held out his hand. "Good work. Give it here and we'll rip it."

Anders handed him the drive and Richard immediately spotted the blood stains. He looked with concern at Anders. "What's this?"

"The price was dear."

Richard gave a sober nod and put it in his pocket.

"You'll be happy to know that Rudy found no further instances of mismatched DNA," Conrad said with uncharacteristic enthusiasm.

"He's sure?"

"Positive," said Conrad. "He's been a busy boy. We've been in touch with the families. There will be compensation, but nothing we can't handle. No one wants to press the issue or see it go public."

"Talk about dodging a bullet," Richard offered.

"Did the CDC ever say why the mothers didn't have symptoms too?"

"Yes," said Conrad. "Let me see if I have this right. The virus was coded to join with valine—something."

"It's one of the essential amino acids. You body doesn't make it, you have to get it from your diet," Anders responded. "It's present in mother's milk."

"Right," said Conrad. "Thierre said that once the virus connected with valine it was able to avoid the antiviral lipids in mother's milk and penetrate the baby's cells and replicate."

Anders' jaw dropped. He turned a small circle and then looked at them in disbelief. "That's incredible. She created a time bomb. The virus could not activate for nine months until the baby took its mother's milk."

"She was a damn genius," Richard said. Both men gave him a stunned look.

Conrad's office door opened suddenly. The three men turned to the sound and saw Torsloff and Keeler barge into the room.

"You again!" Conrad barked. "You're worse than yellow-jackets at a nude picnic."

"National security, Mister Hughes," Keeler volunteered.

"Oh bullshit," Conrad couldn't conceal his disgust. "Your agency hides behind that smoke screen every chance it gets. What are you doing here?"

Torsloff eyed Anders. "We want the doctor to tell us about his adventure in the Middle East."

Anders couldn't believe it. His voice rose. "What? I just got back."

"You met Zaafir Ibrahim," Torsloff continued. "Bad man. An agent for the Pakistani intelligence service. Once helped bin Laden."

"A terrorist?" Anders was still behind the curve.

"No, just a very rich man," said Torsloff. "You might even say, an uber-terrorist. He employs a cadre of scientists to develop new weapons, which he sells to the highest bidder."

"I don't know what to say," replied Anders.

"You brought back a hard drive."

Now Anders was truly dumbfounded. Even Rahman didn't

know he had it.

"Jesus, how did—"

Keller cut him off. "We want it."

Conrad stepped in. "Soon as we find what we need to cure our patients."

"Doctor," Keeler insisted.

Torsloff held up a hand to Keeler. "Look, We've wanted this man for years. There's a chance you could destroy valuable evidence. We can't let you do that."

"And we have sick children." Anders blood was boiling. "The disk has the information we need to cure them. Your terrorists can wait their turn."

"Sorry, Doctor," Torsloff commanded. "National Security. I wish we could oblige."

Conrad saw it was useless. He turned to Richard. "Richard."

Richard took the drive from his pocket and handed it to Torsloff. The agents headed for the door without a word of thanks.

Richard turned to Anders. "Doesn't matter. I'd guess that it's encrypted with algorithms the NSA won't break anytime soon."

"I doubt that," Keeler said over his shoulder.

Anders wanted to beat them senseless. His heart was in his throat. How could they have known? "What a senseless fucking waste," he shouted as the agents reached the door. At least they closed it behind them.

~

Shelves of medical books lined the study in Anders' home. The gold letters on their spines were set aglow by the Tiffany desk lamp, the only light in the darkened room.

Anders brooded in his armchair. He rested his injured leg on the hassock and used both hands to massage his wound. He stopped long enough to reach for a cup of tea on his desk, not minding that it was cold. He heard the doorbell and, unable to ignore it, struggled to his feet.

"Coming," he shouted from the foyer. He reached the door and pulled it open. He was stunned to see Torsloff standing on the stoop holding the hard disk for him to take.

"Thought you might want this back," the agent said. "We didn't find anything."

Anders was astonished. "You broke the encryption?"

"No problem. But the disk was blank. I doubt it could have helped your patients."

Anders felt himself reach for the disk.

"You know there is blood on that."

Anders glanced at the disk in his hand. "What it cost, Agent Torsloff."

Torsloff seemed to understand. He stepped away from the door. Anders went inside and closed the door. As he limped back to the study, he withdrew his mobile and dialed a number.

"Hello, Richard," he said into the phone. "Torsloff just dropped off the hard drive. Said they cracked the disc, but it was blank."

The earpiece said, "Standard security procedure, Anders. Deny information was ever there."

"So, they could have what we need, but they're not going to cooperate."

"Si, amigo. Looks like you'll have to find another way."

Anders had reached the study. "Bastards. Okay. Thanks." He set the phone on the desk and dropped back into his chair. He scolded himself. *Everything I did, I failed. I followed a trail half way around the world, found the prize yet still came up empty handed, no solution. What now? How can I help my patients? They expect answers. I'm their doctor.*

Then start thinking like a doctor, he told himself. *All right. We know this virus will kill my patients and spread god knows where. We know its origin and its phenotype. But only Theresa knows how it became a monster. She must have left a trail.*

Anders reached for his mobile, dialed, and waited for someone to pick up. A female voice answered in Dutch.

"This is Czajkowska."

He responded in Dutch, his voice full of excitement. "Doctor Czajkowska! This is Anders van der Veer. I need your help. We're running out of time to stop this virus."

Anne switched to English. "Doctor? But we finished. What do you want now?"

Anders switched languages also. "Did Theresa know about viruses from Asia?"

"You are thinking of the Alkhurma Hemorrhagic Fever Virus?" she answered quickly. That surprised Anders.

"You knew?"

"I am guessing. There was a French project to sequence the genome. I recall that she may have worked on it."

He couldn't believe his tunnel vision. "I should have called you sooner. The CDC identified the virus. They don't know how to control it."

"A very sinister plan, now that I think about it," Anders could hear the appreciation in her voice. "Infect babies, let them spread the disease."

"I got the hard drive from her computer."

Now Anne was surprised. "You found her computer?"

"The drive is useless," Anders told her.

"But where—oh no. I'm sorry, this is very disturbing." He heard the emotion swell in her voice, but pressed on.

"Yes, it is. And now we're stuck. You're sure she didn't leave any notes?" He listened to static for a long time, almost asked whether she was still there. When Anne did speak, her voice was thoughtful.

"Theresa backed-up her laptop on my server, but I know she deleted all the files."

"What about backup tapes? Where's the server?"

"Here," Anne said. "At the University. You don't think—it's been over a year."

The excitement he now felt gave Anders hope. "Worth a try."

"Doctor, you push too hard."

Anders nodded his silent agreement and waited.

"Very well. I'll be in the lab in thirty minutes. I'll call when I know something." She hung up. He lowered his mobile and raised his eyes to the ceiling as if giving a thankful prayer.

~

If it wasn't the pain in his thigh that kept Anders awake most of the night, it was the anticipation of Anne's return call. When he finally slogged, bleary-eyed into the CDC temporary lab carrying a sixteen-ounce Starbuck's coffee, he hoped he would be alone. Instead, he met Glick. The CDC administrator sat at the lab bench working on a computer.

"Good morning, Doctor," Glick greeted him.

"You're early," he said.

"Couldn't sleep," Glick offered.

"Me neither. Waiting for a phone call."

"Something to help us along, I hope."

"Too early to tell," said Anders and thought, *too early to even be here*. A knock drew the men's attention to the door. It opened wide revealing Amy dressed in an overcoat and carrying a coffee in one hand.

"Doctor van der Veer," she said. "You disappeared last night before I could give you a message."

He hoped Anne hadn't tried to reach him at his office. "What message?"

Amy had a great smile and Anders saw she was giving him the high beams. "Your car will be here today."

Good, but a letdown in light of all that had happened. "Thanks, Amy."

She pulled the door closed and Glick, who'd been watching the exchange said, "Good news?"

The question forced him to consider all of the messages he could have received. He answered truthfully, "I don't know."

His mobile rang. He grabbed it from his pocket, glanced at the Caller ID, smiled, and held it to his ear. *It's all coming together*, he thought. "Doctor Czajkowska?"

~

Anne regarded the frenzy of activity in her Biology Lab at Delft University with a mixture of disgust and anxiety. Half a dozen technicians worked feverishly at computer screens or hustled around the room issuing instructions, redirecting ethernet cables, and carrying equipment. She plugged one ear with her palm to hear over the commotion.

"Doctor van der Veer," she said.

"Did they recover the files?" Anders asked.

This was embarrassing. "We found Theresa's backups, but when we tried to extract the files, our system crashed."

"What?" she heard his surprise.

"Her directory released a program that disabled our servers and the entire network is down."

"Uh-oh," Anders said.

She watched a technician remove the case from one of her computers and prepare to disassemble the interior cabling. "No one can work. The director is furious."

"It wasn't your fault," Anders sounded sympathetic.

"That little bitch! How could I have been so gullible?"

"Not just you—" he started to say. Anne cut him off.

"I must go. Sorry, Doctor, that I cannot help you."

~

Anders closed his mobile, saw that Glick had been watching, heard him say, "No good, eh?"

Anders stared right through the CDC doctor. His mind raced. *Amazing*, he thought. She must have known someone would come after her files and booby trapped the backups. Every trail he followed had led to a dead end. She had neutralized the knowledge of everyone who knew her.

"Doctor? You okay?" he heard Glick ask.

Suddenly, Glick came into focus.

"Where did they sequence the Alkhurma virus?" he asked.

Glick took the question in stride, turned to the computer, and tapped the keyboard.

"Was it France?" Anders thought about the photo of Theresa in Parween's house. Hadn't he said France?

Glick glanced at him with mild surprise. "Yes, there is a citation here for 2001."

"Theresa studied in France," Anders felt his excitement return.

Glick read the screen. "There are several names on this paper."

"She was in Marseilles." It was coming back to him

Glick read the screen again. "Yes. François Reynaud, professor of microbiology at the Université de la Méditerranée in Marseilles."

Anders smiled. "Got his number there?"

$\sim$

Doctor Reynaud knew he had left tomorrow's lecture notes for his morning class on his desk. He pushed from his mind the reoccurring thought that he was going senile and strode down the corridor. He slid the key into the lock of his tiny office in the Biology Department of Université de la Méditerranée. There were the notes. Just as he had thought.

Reynaud stepped to the desk, retrieved the papers, and filed them in his opened briefcase. Case in one hand, coat over one arm, he turned toward the door just as his phone announced that he wasn't done for the day. He stopped, checked at his watch, and reluctantly answered.

"Reynaud," he said into the mouthpiece. Then, "Oui, English is okay."

The professor listened to his caller explain himself and quickly realized that the discussion would not be brief. He placed his satchel and topcoat on his desk and walked around to his chair. As he sat down he heard a name that brought a big smile to his face. He leaned back as memories flooded his imagination.

"Theresa? Oh yes," he told the caller. "Such a beautiful girl! And so talented."

As he listened some more, he thought he was beginning to

understand his caller's intentions.

"Yes, she worked on that project," he said, paused and then sat forward in his chair. "She wrote computer programs to classify various parts of the genome."

What did this man want? So many questions. "I do not remember that," he said after a while. After a few seconds he shook his head. "No. Nothing special."

The questions had become tiresome. Bored, he grabbed a pen and twirled it between two fingers.

Suddenly the caller caught his attention and he sat upright. "Ah, Doctor. Very good question. Just let me have a look."

Reynaud put down the phone, reached over to a file cabinet, and pulled open a drawer. His fingers walked methodically along a row of folders until they found the one he wanted and removed it. The professor spread the file on the desk, extracted a document, and picked up the phone.

"I have it." His voice was triumphant. "She made an elective study, completely voluntary, to silence a part of the genome of the Alkhurma Virus to inhibit replication. It was very original, very clever for the time."

He leafed through the folder while he waited for the caller to respond.

"Well, yes, I suppose." He stuck out his lower lip. "If you know how to stop replication, you must also know to accelerate it."

In response to the caller, Reynaud picked up the paper and counted the pages. "Yes, I can. Would you please give me your fax number? It is eighteen pages."

~

Anders could barely contain his smile. He lowered his mobile and stared at Glick. "You realize I went half way around the world looking for an answer I just got in one phone call."

Glick studied him, seeming to gather his thoughts. "Not really, Doctor. The answer was hidden. Without the journey you wouldn't have known about Dr. Reynard, or where he worked, or the question that would let him unlock the puzzle. No. Your trip was necessary. Congratulations."

~

Anders stood in the Sick Ward between two beds that each held a Davidson twin. He leaned over and stroked the hair of the baby in front of him. He watched Rebecca, one of his nurses, inject a solution into the child's arm. The baby cried when Rebecca swabbed alcohol on her arm.

Anders turned around to face the Davidsons sitting on the other bed. They appeared relieved and relaxed.

"What an amazing turnaround," James said.

"Her body is already producing antibodies. The virus will not spread to other cells," Anders explained.

"I didn't think you could do it," Rose turned and regarded her husband. Anders took comfort in the grateful emotions that flowed between them.

When it seemed like they would overtake Rose, he said softly. "Rose?"

She turned to him with tears running down her face. "I never thought I'd hear myself say it, but thank you, Doctor. I couldn't bear it if they didn't get well. I carried them for nine months. I love them. They're my babies and no lab test can tell me different."

Anders was relieved. "You're welcome, Rose. It was a combined effort." He turned to Jim and gave him a sincere smile. "I should have anticipated mistakes in our lab. I'm sorry I didn't."

Rose leaned over to console the crying baby. James picked up the other twin, held him tenderly, and gave Anders a grateful look.

Anders stepped away to let the parents have their moment. Rebecca stood beside him and they observed the parents before walking toward the door.

"How's the CDC coming along?" Rebecca asked.

"Thanks to the paper from Marseilles, they have the location of the gene. They know exactly what to do. With any luck they'll be out of here tomorrow."

"They discovered what she did?"

"Yes," he stopped and looked at her. "She isolated a gene in the virus, cut it with an enzyme, and inserted foreign DNA into that site. It destroyed the ability of the gene's product, a protein, to function in its normal way, but allowed it to develop another protein that gave the virus an ability to do more harm. The CDC was able to silence the foreign gene."

He watched Rebecca's reaction and decided she understood. She nodded back toward Rose. "That poor family."

This surprised Anders. "Oh I don't know. I think they are very lucky. More than most."

Epilogue

Ibrahim's eyes searched the bleak Parisian dawn. Grey fog swallowed the dreary path winding through the Groupe Hospitalier Pitié-Salpêtriére. A double row of lamps overhead did little to illuminate his journey.

He had grown accustomed to the bandage around his neck, though he objected to the way its stark white clashed with the rest of his elegant attire. At least it would not trouble him much longer. He extended a cold hand and nudged the wheel chair through the winter morning.

Not so for the woman sitting motionless in the rolling seat, staring into the drizzle with empty eyes, the bandages around her head framing her beautiful face. He could never forgive himself for her injury any more than he could forget the words in his head: "Today, you rule everything; tomorrow, nothing."

Ibrahim could not see Theresa's face and missed the moment, only seconds, when fire and determination flashed in her eyes. For him, they would always be empty. So he pushed and they receded into the mist.